# Acupuncture and Moxibustion

P9-DVV-071

*By the same author*

**Le Diagnostic en Médecine Chinoise**
B. Auteroche, P. Navailh
1983, 368 pages, 39 illustrations,
16 black and white plates, 12 colour photographs,
Reprinted 1985, 1988.

**Acupuncture en Gynécologie et Obstétrique**
B. Auteroche, P. Navailh, P. Maronnaud, E. Mullens
Preface by Professor Wang Shanxi,
President of Lian Qiao University, Beijing.
1986, 308 pages.

Neither the publishers nor the author will be liable for any loss or
damage of any nature occasioned to or suffered by any person acting
or refraining from acting as a result of reliance on the material
contained in this publication.

*For Churchill Livingstone:*

*Publisher:* Mary Law
*Project Editor:* Dinah Thom
*Editorial Co-ordination:* Editorial Resources Unit
   *Copy Editor:* Ruth Swan
   *Indexer:* Jill Halliday
*Design:* Design Resources Unit
*Production Controller:* Nancy Henry
*Sales Promotion Executive:* Hilary Brown

# Acupuncture and Moxibustion
## A Guide to Clinical Practice

**B. Auteroche**
**G. Gervais**
**M. Auteroche**
**P. Navailh**
**E. Toui-Kan**

*Translated by* **ORAN KIVITY** B. Ac (MIROM)

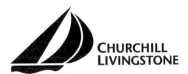
**CHURCHILL LIVINGSTONE**

EDINBURGH LONDON NEW YORK OXFORD PHILADELPHIA ST LOUIS SYDNEY TORONTO 1998

CHURCHILL LIVINGSTONE
An imprint of Elsevier Limited

© Maloine S. A. Editeur 1989

This translation of Pratique des Aiguilles et de la
Moxibustion First edition is published by arrangement with Les
Editions Maloine, Paris.
English edition © Longman Group UK Limited 1992
English edition © Harcourt Brace and Company Limited 1998
English edition © Elsevier Limited 2004

All rights reserved. No part of this publication may be reproduced,
stored in a retrieval system, or transmitted in any
form or by any means, electronic, mechanical,
photocopying, recording or otherwise, without either
the prior permission of the publishers or a licence
permitting restricted copying in the United Kingdom
issued by the Copyright Licensing Agency,
90 Tottenham Court Road, London W1T 4LP.
Permissions may be sought directly from Elsevier's
Health Sciences Rights Department in Philadelphia, USA:
phone: (+1) 215 238 7869, fax: (+1) 215 238 2239,
e-mail: healthpermissions@elsevier.com. You may also
complete your request on-line via the Elsevier Science
homepage (http://www.elsevier.com), by selecting
'Customer Support' and then 'Obtaining Permissions'.

First English edition 1992
  Reprinted 1996
  Reprinted 1998

Transferred to digital printing 2004

ISBN 0 443 04556 9

**British Library of Cataloguing in Publication Data**
A catalogue record for this book is available from the British
Library.

**Library of Congress Cataloging in Publication Data**
A catalog record for this book is available from the Library
of Congress.

**ELSEVIER
SCIENCE**
your source for books,
journals and multimedia
in the health sciences
**www.elsevierhealth.com**

The
publisher's
policy is to use
**paper manufactured
from sustainable forests**

Produced by Addison Wesley Longman Singapore Pte Ltd
Printed and bound by Antony Rowe Ltd, Eastbourne

Zhen Jiu Lin Chuang Cao Zuo
**Acupuncture and Moxibustion**
A Guide to Clinical Practice
Calligraphy by Zhou Hai Ting

针灸临床操作

# Preface to the French edition

Acupuncture is easy to learn; it is the techniques of Reinforcing and Reducing which are difficult to master.

Old medical saying from Shandong province.

The treatment of disease with *Acupuncture and Moxibustion* must take into account several parameters, all of which are indispensable. These are:

1. Developing a clinical picture (Zheng) of the state of the patient with the help of information gathered through the four diagnostic techniques,
2. Finding a group of points in harmony with the therapeutic principle to be put into practice,
3. Correctly stimulating these points by acupuncture or moxibustion.

In the West the first two parameters have been known for some time. The techniques of manipulating the needles, however, have hardly been taught, if at all. Although the practice of needle manipulation has not fallen into disuse in China, as certain westerners would have it, little has been published about acupuncture technique. This is because the student is trained through lengthy apprenticeship during which he repeatedly observes and emulates his teacher's movements. Many works and publications emphasise, however, the importance of needle technique in the therapeutic result and take into account experiments with obtaining and moving Qi, raising and lowering the temperature at the points and the sensations of warmth and cold experienced by the patient (for example, the numerous papers presented at the Second National Symposium of Acupuncture and Moxibustion held in Beijing in August 1984).

This book seeks, as much as possible, to remedy the lack of precision in our knowledge of techniques used in acupuncture and moxibustion. The following method will help the acupuncturist acquire manual skills leading to greater therapeutic effectiveness.

It consists of:

- a description of the tools of the trade and instructions on how to make some of them;
- exercises aimed at giving strength and suppleness to hands and fingers;
- in-depth learning of needle insertion and manipulation techniques, from the simplest to the most complex;
- the study of moxibustion and the use of other types of needles (triangular, cutaneous, long, fire and paediatric), cupping, and manual techniques (pushing and rolling, friction, acupressure);
- a series of Qi Gong exercises (Qi Gong means working on the Qi), daily practice will help the acupuncturist to strengthen the Qi of the organs (Zang-fu) and sharpen his sensory perceptions, in particular his tactile sensitivity;
- a programme of in-depth training spread over a 10-month period.

Each needle or moxibustion technique presented is followed by practical advice on its use: indications and contraindications, the principal ailments it can treat, and examples of point combinations appropriate to the particular manipulation.

The style of needle insertion shown here is not the only one which can be used. The Chinese offer succinct descriptions of several others, each important in its own way, but to master these properly would require a very lengthy apprenticeship.

Our method has several advantages:

● It specifies the respective role of each hand during insertion, thus achieving painless penetration as well as great precision in locating the tip of the needle exactly on the point. It ensures that once the needle has been placed over the point there is no risk of the tip slipping out of position as it is inserted. Errors due to inexact placement of the needle are thus minimised at the moment of insertion.

● It explains how the right hand should hold the needle. This grip is of such importance that a whole section has been devoted to it.

● It illustrates the distinction between active and passive movements. These two movements are complementary and opposed at one and the same time, ensuring correct manipulation.

● The acupuncturist who masters the insertion techniques and the various manipulations taught in this book will easily be able to perform any complex needle technique required, even if he has only a description to go on and has never practised it before.

The importance of obtaining Qi before any manipulation of the needle takes place, and the relation between propagation of Qi and the success of treatment have led us to devote a chapter to the various Qi sensations felt by patient and practitioner alike. Also included are the methods most likely to encourage the arrival of Qi, maintain it and move it once it has been obtained.

Finally, there are two essential concepts to reiterate which, although not further developed here, are the foundations on which this book rests:

● Acupuncture and moxibustion, which together are the principal therapeutic method of external Chinese medicine, use three procedures: Reinforcing (Bu), Reducing (Xie), and Reinforcing and Reducing equally (Ping Bu Ping Xie). These three techniques incorporate the classical Eight Principles of treatment (Ba Fa):

— Reinforcing with needles or moxa consists of the principles of 'Strengthening (Bu)' and 'Warming (Wen)'.
— Reducing includes the principles of 'Inducing Sweating (Han)', 'Inducing Vomiting (Tu)', 'Inducing Catharsis (Xia)',

'Clearing (Qing)', and 'Catalysing (Xiao)'.
— Reinforcing and Reducing equally consists of 'Balancing'.

● The action of the point used varies according to the needle technique selected. For example, in the case of Zusanli ST 36:

— Reinforcing strengthens the Spleen, promotes the Stomach, tonifies the Centre, promotes Qi (Jian Pi Yang Wei, Bu Zhong Yi Qi).
— Reinforcing and adding moxa or reinforcing with the complex manipulation 'Lighting the fire on the mountain' warms and tonifies the Spleen and Stomach (Wen Bu Pi Wei).
— Reducing harmonises the Stomach, opens the intestines, dispels Phlegm and moves stagnation (He Wei Tong Chang, Qu Tang Dao Zhi).
— Reducing then adding moxa, or reducing then adding the complex manipulation 'Lighting the fire on the mountain' warms the Stomach, moves stagnation, warms and transforms Cold and Damp (Wen Wei Dao Zhi, When Hua Han Shi).

We would like to express our gratitude firstly to Doctor Li Tian-yuan, keeper of the orthodox knowledge and thinking of Chinese Medicine, for his concern, his rectitude and the quality of his teaching. We would also like to thank:

— Doctors Eric Mullens and Pierre Maronnaud who were kind enough to take on the role of Candide while revising this text.
— Monsieur Jean-François Ramirez, whose artistic skill provided the vibrant, aesthetic and precise drawings illustrating the essential points of this method.

Finally, we would like to thank all those acupuncturists who encouraged us to persevere in our task with their positive attitude and enquiries. It is our hope that this book will answer some of their questions.

We crave our readers' forgiveness for any errors and omissions which they may find in this text. We should be most grateful for any suggestions or criticisms which would enable us to improve this work.

# Contents

# Using the filiform needle (Hao Zhen)

# 1. The filiform needle: Introduction (Hao Zhen)

The needle most commonly used in acupuncture has been perfected from a description of the seventh of the nine kinds of ancient needle described in Chapter 1 of the *Ling Shu:*

Each of the nine needles differs in both name and form:

1. – Chan needle (arrow-shaped), 1.6 cun long,
2. – Yuan needle (round), 1.6 cun long,
3. – Di needle (blunt), 3.5 cun long,
4. – Feng needle (sharp-edged), 1.6 cun long,
5. – Pi needle (sword-shaped), 4 cun long, 0.25 cun wide,
6. – Yuan-Li (round and sharpened), 1.6 cun long,
7. – Hao needle (fine, like a strand of hair), 3.6 cun long,
8. – Chang needle (long), 7 cun long,
9. – Da needle (big), 4 cun long.

1. – The Chan needle is used for external perverse influences which have penetrated into the body. The tip of this needle is in the shape of an arrow. It is used at the level of the skin.

2. – The Yuan needle is rounded at the tip and is used for shallow massage.

3. – The Di needle has a blunt tip which does not penetrate the skin. Its effect is only on the surface.

4. – The Feng needle is sharp-edged and is used for bleeding the acupuncture points.

5. – The Pi needle has a sharp sword-like tip. It is used for opening the skin to discharge pus.

6. – The Yuan Li needle has a sharp, thick and rounded tip. It is used in the treatment of acute disease.

7. – The Hao needle is very fine. It is used for obstruction, articular pain and paralysis. It can be left in place in the body.

8. – The Chang needle is long, fine and very sharp. It is used for paralysis and obstruction.

9. – The Da needle is round and thick with a sharp tip. It is used in the treatment of articular swellings and to drain fluid from swollen joints. (Figs 1.1, 1.2)

The Hao needle, i.e. the filiform needle, is also known as the fine or capillary needle. It comes in different metals: gold, silver, alloy or steel. Gold, silver and alloy needles are expensive, soft and difficult to maintain. The 'aura' of Yin and Yang which they possess does not compensate for these drawbacks. The needle most commonly used is made of stainless steel. This does not rust and has a good resistance to heat. It is also quite flexible. Filiform needles come in different lengths and diameters.

***Dimensions***. Length is expressed either in cun or in millimetres. One cun or Chinese inch is equal to 3.33 centimetres or 1.31 inches. Diameter is expressed either by gauge number or in millimetres.

| | Length | | | | | | | | |
|---|---|---|---|---|---|---|---|---|---|
| *Body* | | | | | | | | | |
| cun | 0.5 | 1 | 1.5 | 2 | 2.5 | 3 | 4 | 5 | 6 |
| mm | 15 | 25 | 40 | 50 | 65 | 75 | 100 | 125 | 150 |
| *Handle* (mm) | | | | | | | | | |
| Long | 25 | 35 | 40 | 40 | 40 | 40 | 55 | 55 | 55 |
| Medium | — | 30 | 35 | 35 | — | — | — | — | — |
| Short | 20 | 25 | 25 | 30 | 30 | 30 | 40 | 40 | 40 |
| | Diameter | | | | | | | | |
| Gauge (No.) | 26 | 27 | 28 | 29 | 30 | 31 | 32 | 34 | |
| mm | 0.45 | 0.42 | 0.38 | 0.34 | 0.32 | 0.30 | 0.28 | 0.23 | |

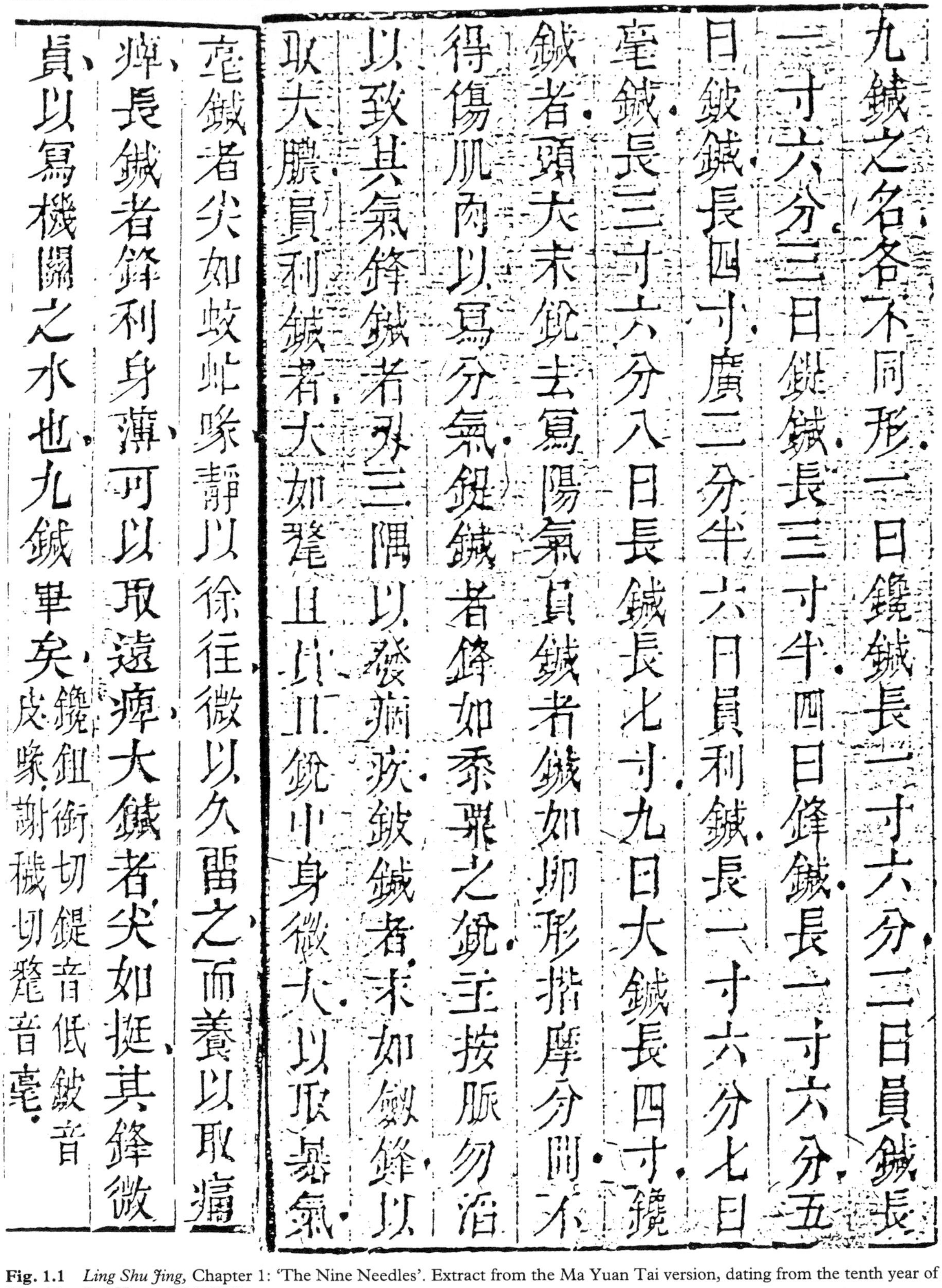

九鍼之名各不同形一曰鑱鍼長一寸六分二曰員鍼長
一寸六分三曰鍉鍼長三寸半四曰鋒鍼長一寸六分五
曰鈹鍼長四寸廣二分半六曰員利鍼長一寸六分七日
毫鍼長三寸六分八日長鍼長七寸九日大鍼長四寸鑱
鍼者頭大末銳去寫陽氣員鍼者鍼如卵形揩摩分間不
得傷肌肉以寫分氣鍉鍼者鋒如黍粟之銳主按脈勿陷
以致其氣鋒鍼者刃三隅以發痼疾鈹鍼者末如劍鋒以
取大膿員利鍼者大如氂且圓且銳中身微大以取暴氣
毫鍼者尖如蚊虻喙靜以徐往微以久留之而養以取痛
痺長鍼者鋒利身薄可以取遠痺大鍼者尖如挺其鋒微
員以寫機關之水也九鍼畢矣 皮喙謝穢切鑱鑱音毫
鈹鈕衛切鍉音低鈹音

**Fig. 1.1** *Ling Shu Jing*, Chapter 1: 'The Nine Needles'. Extract from the Ma Yuan Tai version, dating from the tenth year of Nian Hao Rui Huang Ti (1806).

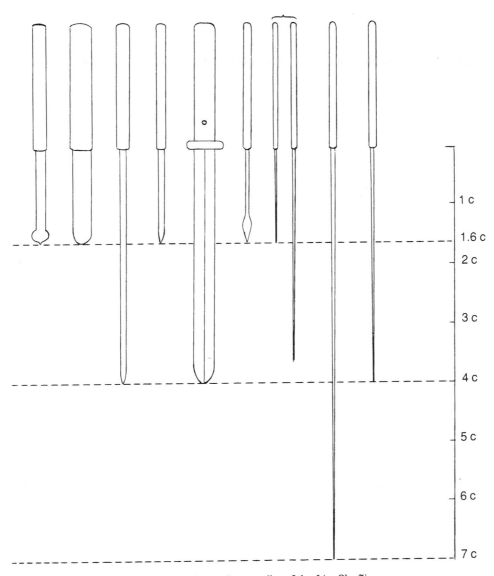

**Fig. 1.2**   The nine ancient needles of the *Ling Shu Jing*.

0.5 cun needles are generally used only for children or for pricking points on the face or head. 1.5 and 2 cun needles are commonly used for points on the body or limbs. 3 and 4 cun needles are good for points in the muscular areas of the body, like Huantiao GB 30, and for joining points, for example linking Hegu LI 4 to Houxi SI 3, or Yanglingquan GB 34 to Yinlingquan Sp 9. 30 and 32 gauge needles are the most commonly used. 26 or 28 gauge needles are good when bleeding or strong reducing is required.

*Only stainless steel needles are recommended.*
- *During training — length 1.5 cun (body 40 mm, handle 40 mm), 34 gauge (diameter 0.23 mm).*
- *In clinical practice — 34 gauge, but with varying lengths: 1 cun (body 25 mm, handle 25 mm), 1.5 cun, 3 cun (body 75 mm, handle 75 mm).*

The filiform needle consists of five parts: tip, body, root, handle and tail (Fig. 1.3).

**The tip** should not be too sharp. On the contrary it is described as being slightly rounded, 'like

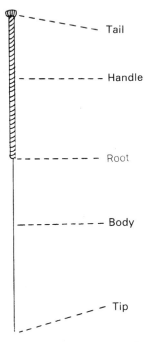

**Fig. 1.3** The filiform needle.

a fir needle, so it moves the blood vessels out of the way'.

Whilst the needle is being manipulated and during everyday maintenance, a knock can bend the sharpened tip into a hook. To ensure that the tip is in good condition the following methods can be used:

*Before sterilisation:* Hold the needle by the handle between thumb and index finger of the right hand. Rest the tip of the needle on the pad of the middle finger of the left hand. Rotate the needle with your right thumb and index finger. An unpleasant catching sensation on the pad of your left middle finger indicates that the tip is in bad condition.

*After sterilisation:* Rotate the tip of the needle on a sterile cotton wool swab. If the point is not true it will get caught up in the cotton wool fibres.

To repair and sharpen the tip use an emery cloth or a fine oilstone. Rub the tip crosswise to give it the desired roundness.

**The body** should be straight, flexible, firm and sturdy and the same diameter all the way down. If the body is bent it can be repaired using one of the following methods:

1. With your left hand hold the handle of the needle with the tip pointing vertically upwards. Grip the root of the needle tightly between thumb and index finger of your right hand and slowly lift them towards the tip whilst sliding the needle downwards in the opposite direction to the bend in the body.

2. If the curvature is very pronounced, put the needle down flat on the edge of a table. With your right hand, press the root of the needle against the table with a hardwood ruler then slowly withdraw the needle with the left.

**The root** is where the handle joins the body. This is a delicate area which should be examined very closely for signs of wear, corrosion and rust, indicating that the needle may break.

**The handle** is a tightly wound coil of wire. It should be sturdy and able to withstand being twisted. The length of the handle of the filiform needle should be proportionate to the length of the body. In our opinion they should be equal in length. If the handle of the needle is longer than the body then the two will not be counterbalanced after insertion; the handle will tend to lean over to one side causing difficulties when manipulating the needle.

If the handle is much shorter than the body it will also cause difficulties during manipulation, particularly if it is necessary to rotate the needle.

### Care and sterilisation of needles

The acupuncturist has a duty to bring the utmost care to the quality and maintenance of his needles:

— The quality of the metal and the technique of manufacture used determine the dynamic properties of the needle, and need to be taken into account to achieve the best results.

— Proper maintenance is of the utmost importance. The body of the needle must be absolutely straight and the tip should not be blunted or hooked. It is important to look out for such flaws during cleaning, sterilisation and use. The needles must be checked regularly so they do not present any risk to the patient or cause additional pain. Needles should not be used unless the acupuncturist is satisfied that they are in perfect condition.

— It is essential to sterilise the needles after

each use. According to French standards (AFNOR NFT 72101, Journal Officiel, February 4th 1981) acupuncturists must:

1. Rinse the needles in disinfectant and detergent solution, following the directions of and conforming to AFNOR standards.

2. Rinse the needles in fresh water.

3. Sterilise the needles with dry heat at 170°C for one hour.

Acupuncturists may offer a choice to patients:

- Sterilised needles.
- Sterilised needles reserved for use on one patient only. This involves extra administration for the practitioner.
- Disposable needles. This is an interesting alternative to the other two options, but significant advances need to be made both in price and in the quality of the materials. Those disposable needles which we have used have not been altogether satisfactory.

## Translator's note

British Council for Acupuncture guidelines (1989) recommend washing needles in soap and water before sterilising. Sterilisation should be either by autoclave or by dry heat, for the following times:

|  | Temperature in degrees Centigrade | Minimum holding time in minutes (when required temperature has been achieved) |
|---|---|---|
| Autoclave (preferred method) | 121 | 15 |
|  | 126 | 10 |
|  | 134 | 3 |
| Oven dry heat (metal objects only) | 160 | 45 |
|  | 170 | 18 |
|  | 180 | 8 |
|  | 190 | 2 |

# 2. Inserting the filiform needle

*Su Wen*, Chapter 25:

It is the physician's choice whether to use deep or shallow insertion, whether to make the energy come from far away or nearby, but at all times he must maintain total concentration and act as if he were standing on the edge of an abyss or holding back a tiger.

There are two factors determining correct needle insertion:

- the strength exerted by the fingers and the suppleness of the wrist,
- the way in which the needle is placed on the point.

Most training procedures start with practice first on folded paper, then on a cotton ball wrapped in cloth. This is a sound approach and a useful way to start. Developing correct technique, however, requires a gradual and regular programme of training. The hand, wrist and fingers must be strengthened and made more supple, and proper needle insertion technique must be acquired.

The method outlined in the first part of this chapter describes a way of realising these two objectives gradually. The second part provides necessary advice to the acupuncturist for use in daily practice.

## A. BASIC TRAINING

### 1. Practising on folded paper

Fold some sheets of soft paper (kitchen roll, tissues, etc.) into a square 6 cm wide and 2 cm thick. Bind them all together with string, marking out a space in the centre like a well (Jing).

Hold the paper square loosely in your left hand. Hold a 1.5 cun needle by the handle between thumb, index and middle finger of your right hand. Keeping the needle perpendicular to the paper, thrust it in with a push from the fingers and wrist of your right hand. As you push down, rotate the needle alternately in both directions through an angle of about 180° (Fig. 2.1).

When the needle has passed through the paper, change position and start again.

### 2. Practising on a cotton ball

When you have gained flexibility and strength and can easily insert the needle into paper, make a cotton ball on which to practise handling the needle. Take some material, soak it, wring it out and leave it to dry. Wrap this up with string to make a ball 7 or 8 cm in diameter and cover the whole thing tightly in strong cotton (Fig. 2.2).

## B. TRAINING PROGRAMME

There are two parts to this training programme: a set of general exercises designed to develop the strength and flexibility of the wrists and fingers, and specific exercises with the needle.

### Developing the fingers and wrist

#### Ball exercises (Jian Sheng Qiu)

The use of balls as training tools is very old and is mentioned in Chapter 24 of the *Zhuang Zi*, written in the 4th century BC. Exercises involving balls of increasing weight and size help to build strength, stamina and flexibility in both left hand and right.

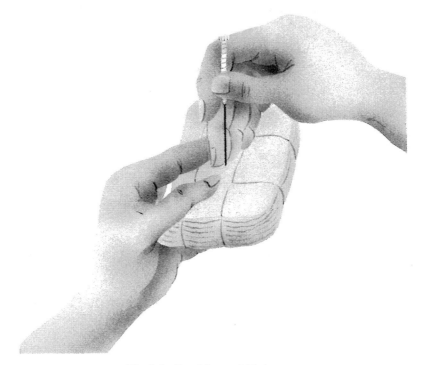

**Fig. 2.1** Practising on folded paper.

These qualities are necessary for:

- the involvement of the left hand in needle insertion,

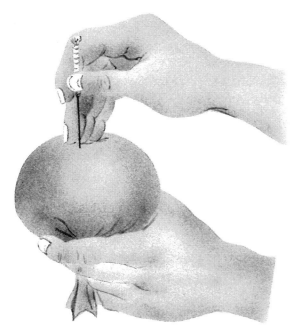

**Fig. 2.2** Practising on a cotton ball.

- manipulating the needle,
- moving muscular structures out of the way to locate the point,
- giving massage (Tui Na).

*Training equipment*

- 2 golf balls (American type)
- 2 round stones of identical size (one size for men, one size for women)
- 2 steel balls of identical size (one size for men, one size for women).

*Position*

Do the exercise sitting down. Sit straight on the edge of a hard chair, knees at right angles and slightly apart, feet firmly on the floor. Before starting, your back should be perfectly straight, shoulders lowered and relaxed. Hold your arms loosely, palms resting on your knees. When one hand is in action, the other remains in place.

Throughout the exercise keep your eyes fixed on your hand and concentrate your mind on performing the movement. The exercise is less

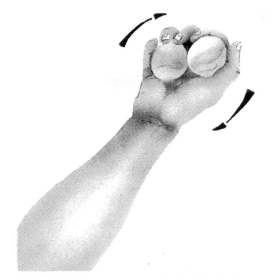

**Fig. 2.3** Turning the balls with the right hand.

effective if you allow yourself to be distracted. It is best to work in silence, without shifting position.

*Rolling the balls*

Always start the exercise with the left hand. Hold the two balls in the palm of your hand, arm slightly extended at 45° to the axis of the body. Rotate the balls anti-clockwise with thumb and fingers, keeping them in motion by using each digit consecutively. Make sure that each finger flexes on the balls in succession. When practising with the right hand, rotate the balls clockwise (Fig. 2.3).

Practise the same exercise consecutively with the golf balls, the round stones and the steel balls, following the timetable outlined in Appendix I.

**NB**: Whatever type of ball is being used, the following points should be observed:

- Whilst turning the balls avoid moving your arm; only your fingers should be moving.
- The balls' circular movement should be as precise and regular as possible.
- Keep the balls in contact all the time, so that they do not bang against each other.
- Do not exceed the recommended times during practice or you may risk developing epicondylitis or tendinitis.

**Stick exercises**

The aim of this exercise is to build up strength in the wrist and fingers. It puts a lot of strain on the elbow so if any cramps or pains develop discontinue the exercise for a while then return to it very gradually.

*Training equipment*

— For women: a stick made of hard wood, 30 cm long, 2.9–3 cm in diameter.
— For men: a stick made of hard wood, 40 cm long, 2.9–3 cm in diameter.

*Method*

*Starting position.* Stand up straight and well balanced, with feet parallel and shoulder-width apart. Start the exercise with the right hand. Hold the stick firmly by one end and let your arm hang down by your body. Your hand should be semi-pronated, i.e. the back of your hand facing the front.

*Stage 1.* Without moving your arm, raise the stick as high as possible, keeping your hand semi-pronated and flexing the elbow slightly if necessary (Fig. 2.4a).

*Stage 2.* With a violent motion thrust the end of the stick forwards, straightening your arm and lifting it to the height of an imaginary opponent's solar plexus.

At the end of this phase your arm should be tensed, hand still semi-pronated, with the stick in perfect alignment with the plane of the inner aspect of the arm (Fig. 2.4b).

*Stage 3.* Supinate the hand and then pull it back forcibly to your nipple, keeping the end of the stick gripped firmly in your palm (Fig. 2.4c).

*Stage 4.* Turn your hand back into semi-pronation and snap it back into position by your leg like a whip.

*Duration of practice.* Allow each stage to flow rhythmically into the next one without pausing. Practise with your right hand first, then your left. Start with 1 minute per hand and increase gradually to a maximum of 5 minutes per hand (see Appendix I).

**Bottle exercises**

This exercise follows on from the previous one.

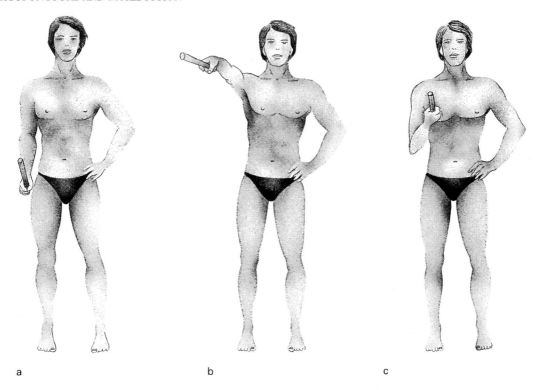

a                                    b                                    c

**Fig. 2.4a–c**  Stick exercise. **a** Stage 1. **b** Stage 2. **c** Stage 3.

*Equipment*

2 plastic 1 litre bottles filled with water. These should have a long neck so that they can be held firmly.

*Starting position*

Stand up straight and well balanced, with feet parallel and shoulder-width apart.

*Method*

Hold a bottle by its neck in each hand and let them hang down by your sides. Without moving your arms raise and lower the bottles slowly and rhythmically, flexing the elbow slightly if necessary.

*Duration of practice*

Start off by practising for 1 minute and increase gradually to a maximum of 5 minutes (see Appendix I).

### Qi Gong exercises

The aim of these exercises is to regulate and strengthen the circulation of blood and energy and to harmonise the functions of the organs. In addition, they enhance the practitioner's sensory abilities, particularly the delicate sensitivity of the fingertips. Regular practice of these exercises is therefore a particularly effective way of acquiring the delicacy of touch necessary for needle manipulation.

Chapter 10 is devoted entirely to detailed descriptions of the five Qi Gong exercise cycles, complete with illustrations.

### Practising with needles

#### Polishing the needle

Buy a 5 × 2.5 cm rectangle of finest grade emery cloth. The type used for finishing the surfaces of model aeroplanes is best.

Make a square by folding the rectangle in half, the rough side of the cloth facing inwards. Place

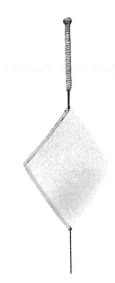

**Fig. 2.5** Polishing the needle: position of needle in paper square.

the square between the thumb and index finger of your left hand with the open edge of the paper facing the palm. Tilt the square upwards from the bottom so it looks like a diamond. Insert the needle through the open side and wedge the body in the upper part of the point of the diamond (Fig. 2.5).

Sit very straight on the edge of a hard chair, knees at right angles and slightly apart, feet parallel and flat on the ground. With your back perfectly straight hold out your left hand level with the sternal notch, so you can see it, keeping the needle vertical.

Move your right wrist slightly outwards so that the first metacarpal is on a straight line drawn from the radial edge of the forearm. Take hold of the needle at the root, holding it between the pads of the thumb and index finger of your right hand. Keep your shoulders lowered and your elbows close to your body.

With your right hand rotate the needle using three fingers, the pad of your thumb against the pads of your middle and index fingers. Rotate the needle anti-clockwise 2 or 3 times by drawing your thumb towards you, keeping the movements smooth. At the same time push the needle downwards approximately 1 cm (Fig. 2.6a). Next pull the needle up whilst rotating it through the same angle in the opposite direction (Fig. 2.6).

**NB**: Throughout the exercise keep your forearms still, elbows close to your body. Only the right hand, leading from the wrist, goes up and down in harmony with the movement of the needle.

Continue raising and lowering the needle for 5 minutes, being careful to keep your concentration firmly on the actions of both hands. During this exercise your concentration on the movements

a                                            b

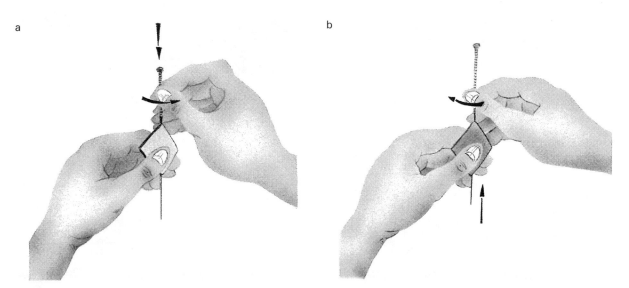

**Fig. 2.6a, b** Polishing the needle. **a** Push the needle downwards, pulling your thumb towards you. **b** Pull the needle up, extending your thumb away from you.

should be absolute, so stop work altogether if you find yourself getting tired.

### Practising on a cushion

#### 1. Making a practice cushion

##### Materials:

- A rectangle of strong fine cotton cloth, tightly woven and uncoloured, measuring approximately 30 cm × 40 cm
- One sheet of pure cotton wool, 20 cm × 50 cm × 3 cm
- A second sheet of pure cotton wool, 20 cm × 40 cm × 1.5 cm
- A 3 m length of pure cotton twine, diameter 2 mm
- Ironing starch (aerosol)
- Sewing needle and thread
- Pins
- Adhesive tape.

##### Instructions:

1. Apply the starch to the twine and leave it to dry, repeating as necessary until it is stiff. Next tie a slipknot with a wide loop at one end.

2. Take the thickest (3 cm) sheet of cotton wool and place the narrow (20 cm) end in front of you on the edge of a table. Starting from this end, roll the cotton wool up as tightly as possible, making sure that the width of the roll stays the same (Fig. 2.7a). Use your little fingers to keep the cotton wool from sticking out at the sides (Fig. 2.7b). Continue until you have a roll roughly 5–6 cm in diameter.

**NB:** Make sure the cotton wool has not been squashed or flattened before use, and do not roll and unroll it too many times.

3. Place the slipknot over one end of the roll and pull it tight. Following the direction in which the cotton wool has been rolled, wind the twine round 7 or 8 times. The twine should hold the cotton wool in position without indenting it too deeply. Fix the twine to the other end of the roll with a half hitch and come back in the opposite direction criss-crossing over the first layer. Fix the twine permanently in place with a knot and cut off the excess.

4. Lay out a dozen pins and the needle and thread. Anchor one end of the piece of cloth to the work surface with adhesive tape. Next place the roll at one end of the second, thinner (1.5 cm) sheet of cotton wool (Fig. 2.7c). Wind the cotton wool tightly around the roll. Use your hands and the weight of your body to stop the cotton wool extending past the edges of the roll (Fig. 2.7d).

a
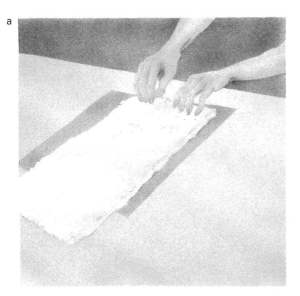

b
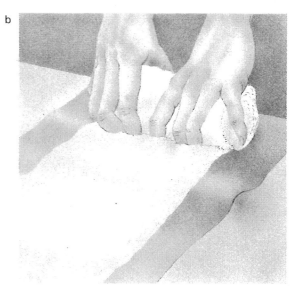

**Fig. 2.7a–b** Making the cushion. **a** Roll the cotton wool up tightly. **b** Use your little fingers to keep the cotton wool from protruding at the sides.

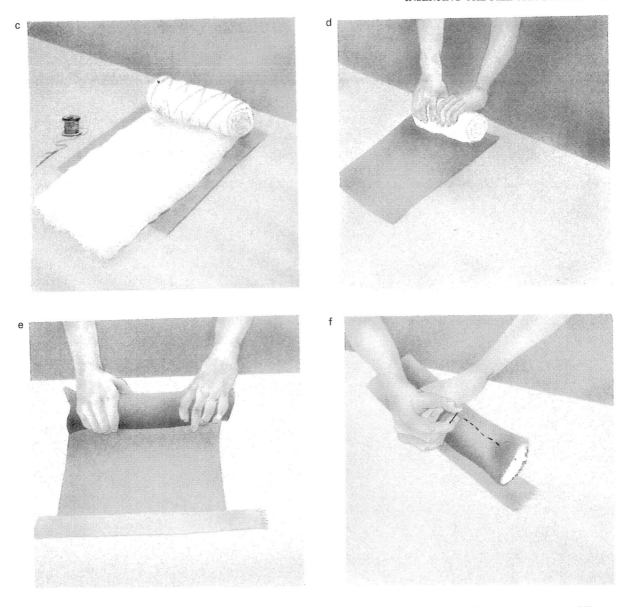

**Fig. 2.7c–f**  **c** Rolling up the second sheet of cotton wool. Note the indentations on the first roll made by the twine. **d** Keep the second roll tightly wound. **e** Wrap the cloth around the cotton wool roll (note the piece of adhesive tape in the foreground, anchoring the free end of the cloth to the work surface). **f** Use pins to hold the cloth in place.

The new roll should be about 7 cm in diameter. Keeping it tightly wound, place it at the narrow end of the square of cloth (Fig. 2.7e). Using your thumbs to grip the cloth, wrap it around the roll, pressing tightly. When the roll has been covered with cloth, pin the overlapping edges together in a straight line. Cut off the excess, but leave enough hem for stitching (Fig. 2.7f).

5. Sew using very small stitches. While sewing make sure that the upper overlap lies flat on the lower overlap, pulling it over to keep the fabric tightly stretched. Use an occasional cross-stitch to strengthen the seam. Do not pierce the cotton wool underneath. Once the length of the roll is sewn up, close off one end with a couple of cross-stitches. Push the roll of cotton wool firmly down

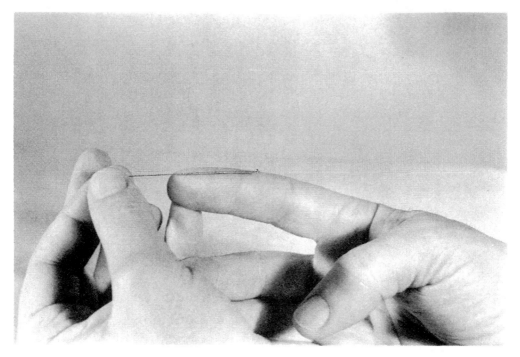

**Fig. 2.8** Holding the needle. Position of the needle on the index finger. Note that the handle rests on the lateral edge of the finger.

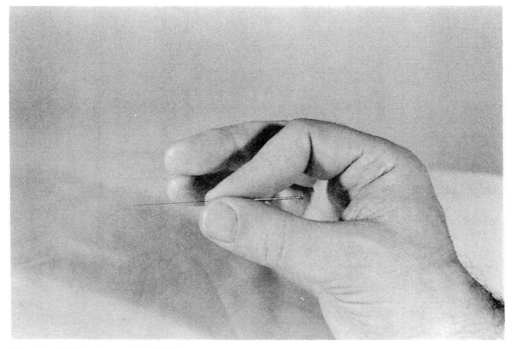

**Fig. 2.9** Holding the needle. Hold the needle at the root between the pads of the thumb and index finger (lateral edge of the index finger and medial edge of the thumb).

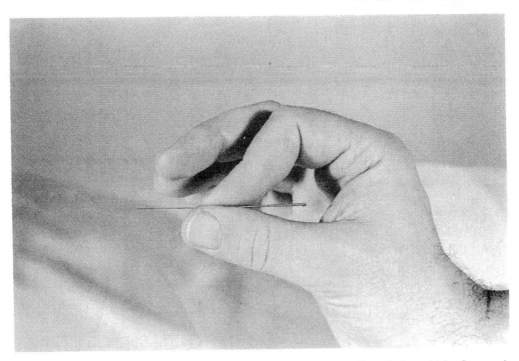

**Fig. 2.10**  Holding the needle. Pull back the index finger. As the proximal interphalangeal joint flexes and the distal phalangeal joint extends, the hand resembles the roof of a house.

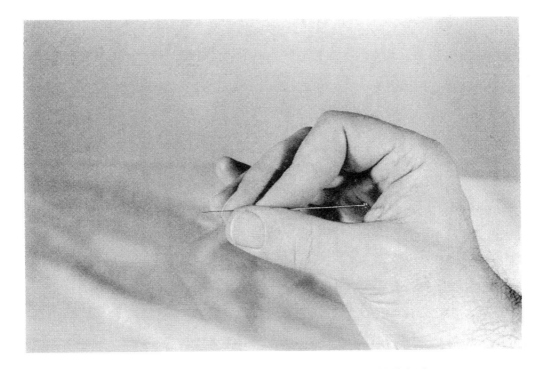

**Fig. 2.11**  Holding the needle. Positioned in this way the fingers look like a bird's beak.

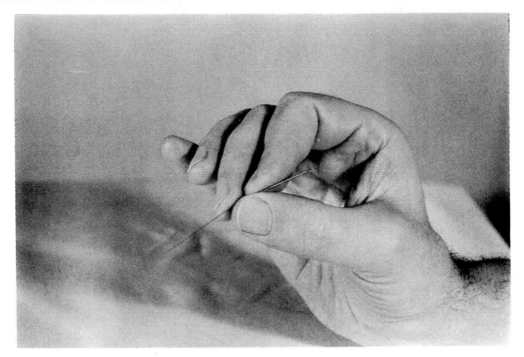

**Fig. 2.12** Alternative method of holding the needle. Compare with Fig. 2.11

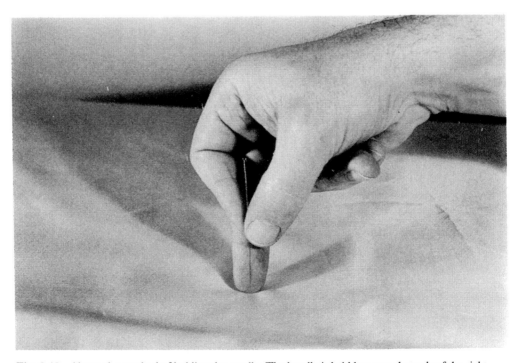

**Fig. 2.13** Alternative method of holding the needle. The handle is held between the pads of the right thumb and index fingers.

inside its case and close off the other end with two more cross-stitches.

This practice cushion (Zhentou) will be used for the study of needle insertion and the different ways of manipulating the needle (these manipulations are all grouped together in Ch. 5).

*2. Perpendicular needle insertion*

Perpendicular needle insertion can be broken down into two stages:

a. holding the needle
b. piercing the skin.

***a. Holding the needle***. The needle is held in the right hand. In China left-handed students are also taught to needle with the right hand, not the left.

Hold the needle at the root between the lateral edge of the pads of thumb and index finger (Figs. 2.8, 2.9). The tip of the needle points forward, and the needle itself is held precisely in the plane of the pincer formed by the thumb and index finger. The thumb is straight. The proximal interphalangeal joint (PIP) of the index finger is flexed whereas the distal interphalangeal joint (DIP) is loosely extended.

Pull back the index finger about 1 cm along the thumb, dragging the needle back with it. The thumb remains completely straight. Increase the flexion of the proximal interphalangeal (PIP) and the extension of the distal interphalangeal (DIP) so the whole thing ends up resembling the roof of a house (Fig. 2.10).

Next, position the pad of the third finger on the body of the needle and apply gentle pressure to give it a slight curvature.

When these three fingers are held in this way the third finger and thumb form a kind of mortise into which the index finger is inserted. They can also be likened to a beak, into which no daylight can penetrate. The tip of the needle projects beyond the third finger by about 1 cm (Fig. 2.11).

The grip on the needle should always be flexible and relaxed. *The fingers should never be tense.*

NB: Many sources describe alternative methods of holding the needle:

— The needle is held by the handle between thumb, index and third finger of the right hand, with the pad of the thumb opposite the gap between index and third finger (Fig. 2.12).

— The needle is held by the handle between pad of thumb and index finger. This method is not for beginners (Fig. 2.13).

— The needle is held by the body, with the pads of index finger and thumb on the lower part of the needle. The tip of the needle projects no more than 1 cm beyond the fingers. This method is used when it is necessary to put the needle in very quickly but it is also the technique for filiform needles 3 cun in length (Fig. 2.14 and see Ch. 7 'Long needle').

***b. Needling***

*Nan Jing*, Chapter 78:

He who knows the needle trusts his left hand; he who is unfamiliar with it trusts his right.

Perpendicular insertion is the first stage of needle

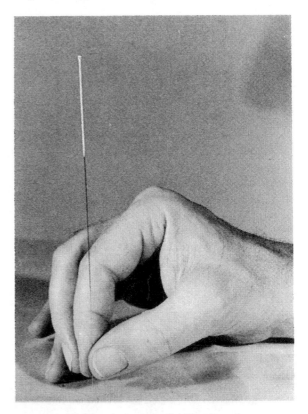

**Fig. 2.14** Holding the long needle. The tip projects no more than 1 cm beyond the fingers.

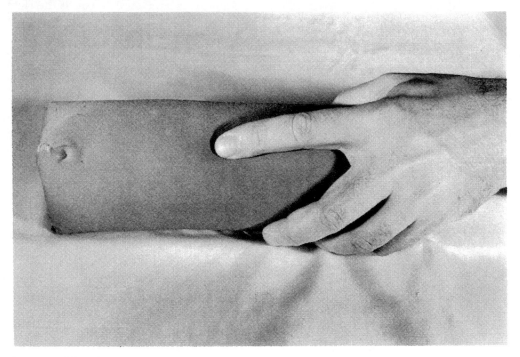

**Fig. 2.15** Tiger claw.

manipulation. It is accomplished by the interaction of left hand and right.

*Role of the left hand.* The left hand lies longitudinally along the axis of the practice cushion, grasping it firmly. The index finger rests on top, marking the point to be needled. In addition, the tip of the index finger pushes down, bracing and holding the skin around the point. All needle manipulations will start off with the left hand in this position, which corresponds to what is known in the classical texts as 'tiger claw' (Fig. 2.15).

The left hand, far from being passive, plays an active role. Not only does it rest on the structures around the point but it exerts a broad grip on the tissues, keeping them firmly in place. At the same time the index finger presses down so any vascular and/or nervous tissue at risk of being punctured is moved out of the way. Immobilising the muscle helps to obtain Qi.

There are variations on the position of the left hand:

— The edge of the left thumbnail is pressed down on the point. Pressure is applied to the point with the second phalanx of index and third fingers to hold the skin in place (Fig. 2.16a).

— With the fingers of the left hand straight the skin is stretched, either between the index and third finger, or between third finger and thumb. This method is used on those places where the skin is loose and flabby (Fig. 2.16b, Fig. 2.17).

— The thumb and index finger pinch the place to be needled, making it stick up. In this case the insertion is horizontal. This method is useful for those places where the surface tissue is thin, e.g. the points on the face (Fig. 2.16c).

*Role of the right hand.* With your left hand holding the cushion firmly, the right hand grasps the needle in the way described above. Sliding along the nail of the third finger, the right hand is brought in from the side to locate the tip of the needle on the point (Fig. 2.18).

Next, using the tip of the third finger as a fulcrum, the right hand lifts up to the vertical and pivots slightly to the left, so that the plane formed by the pincer of index finger to thumb is exactly perpendicular to the plane in which the left index finger lies.

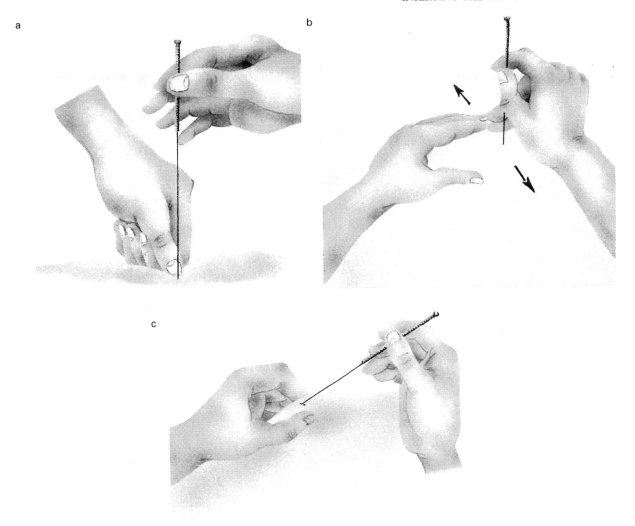

**Fig. 2.16** **a–c** Position of the left hand during insertion. **a** Variation 1; **b** Variation 2; **c** Variation 3.

Note that at the moment when the hand starts to move towards the vertical, the tip of the needle still protrudes from between the fingers by 1 cm. To enable the third finger to provide support for the turn without pushing the needle into the cushion or the skin, the protruding centimetre has to be retracted. As the hand lifts up and pivots, the needle pushes down very gently on the surface of the cloth. This imperceptible pressure is enough to slide it back up between the loosely held thumb and index finger (Fig. 2.19).

*Thus, as the needle is put into place, there is no change at any time in the position of the three fingers described at the start.*

Note that right up to the actual insertion the fingers are never tense when holding the needle. The contact is always flexible and relaxed.

It is from this position that the actual insertion takes place.

*Piercing the skin.* At the moment of penetration the two hands work synergistically. The *Ling Shu* Chapter 1 says, 'The left hand pushes, the right hand inserts'.

To do this the left index finger gives a brief extra push to the surface of the cushion. This comes a fraction of a second before the action of the right hand to mask the insertion of the needle.

This push is instantly followed by the penetration of the needle: at this point the third finger of the right hand increases its pressure on the

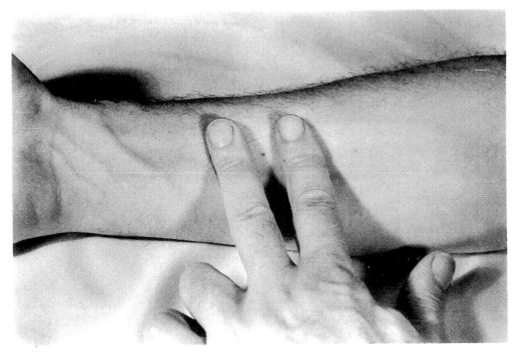

**Fig. 2.17**   Move the index and third fingers apart to stretch the skin.

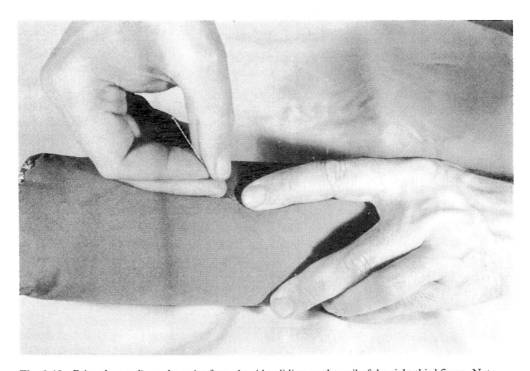

**Fig. 2.18**   Bring the needle to the point from the side, sliding on the nail of the right third finger. Note the position of the needle on the lateral edges of the right index and third fingers.

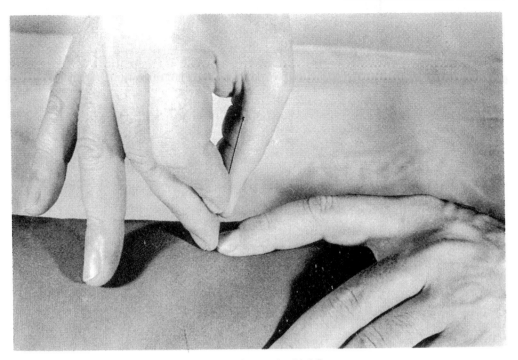

**Fig. 2.19**    Bring the hand to the vertical by pivoting on the third finger.

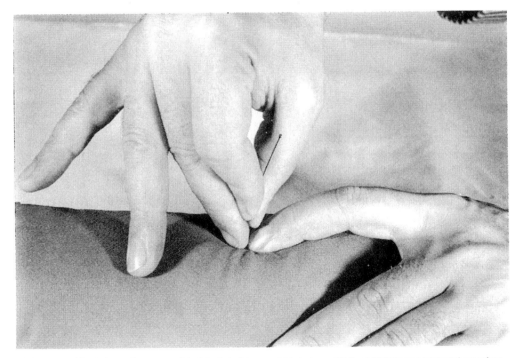

**Fig. 2.20**    'The left hand presses, the right hand inserts.' Note how the four fingers are grouped together, and the creases in the cloth at the moment of insertion (the body of the needle is at right angles to the surface of the cloth). The curve in the needle is a result of the pressure of the fingers.

cushion while at the same time the pincer formed by the right thumb and index finger tenses, pushing the needle in like a piston (Fig. 2.20).

The entire sequence should not result in a heavy and exaggerated push from the fingers. On the contrary, penetration is best achieved with a brisk and rapid movement of index finger and thumb. If the third finger applies the correct pressure as the needle goes in, it exerts a supplementary tension on the underlying tissues, which also helps to make the insertion painless.

At this stage the needle should have penetrated the skin painlessly to a depth of 3–5 mm. Without pausing, push very slowly on the needle twice more, pressing it down like a piston until it is something like 1.2 cm deep. Use all your concentration to perform these movements, bearing in mind the underlying anatomical structures in accordance with the old saying: 'the Shen (spirit) should accompany the tip of the needle in its exploration'.

*Other insertion techniques*

**1. Needle insertion into tough skin.** The needle is inserted through the contraction of the right thumb and index finger. Vibrate the needle in a continuous series of short jolts until it is through the epidermis (practising the fourth Qi Gong exercise will make this technique much easier, see Ch. 10).

Once the needle is through the skin it can be pushed deeper either by the method described in the previous section or by giving it a tiny backwards and forwards rotation until it has reached the desired depth.

**2. Traditional needle insertion.** In the past the iron in the needle was much more rigid than today. With thumb, index and third finger holding the root, it was possible to insert the needle by jolting it skilfully in a continuous series of Yin vibrations (Yin energy corresponds to shaking, Yang energy to thrusting). This series of movements can still be performed today with a filiform needle but only if the practitioner has trained properly in Qi Gong or is well versed in classical needle insertion.

If the 'vibrating' method of insertion is used, it

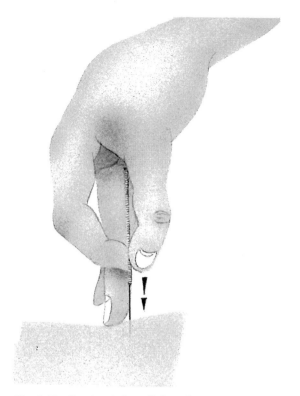

**Fig. 2.21**   One-handed needle insertion.

is necessary to hold the skin tight for the needle. This can be done in several ways:

- stretch the skin between left thumb and index finger,
- stretch the skin with the ulnar edge of the right hand,
- combine the above methods.

**3. One-handed insertion.** The above techniques require the use of both hands. Needling with one hand is possible if the practice of two-handed insertion has been fully mastered.

*Method 1:* The handle is gripped between the pads of index finger and thumb, the third finger extended along the body of the needle. Thumb and index finger are parallel with the handle of the needle.

At the moment of insertion, penetration is achieved by the flexion and extension of the joints of the thumb and index finger. The third finger acts as a guide, and remains anchored to the point (Fig. 2.21).

*Method 2:* The body of the needle is gripped

between the pads of thumb and index finger. At the moment of insertion the tip of the needle and the practitioner's wrist make contact with the patient at the same time. This method of penetration is generally painless. After insertion the practitioner's wrist remains resting on the patient's skin. The thumb and index finger relax their grip on the needle and move upwards, taking hold of it again at the upper end of the body, and then slowly push the needle into the point. This method is good for fairly long needles for use on the points on the lumbar area, buttocks and legs.

## C. GUIDELINES FOR CLINICAL PRACTICE

### Variations in insertion

There are two parameters to take into consideration when inserting the needle:

- angle of insertion
- depth of insertion.

### *Angle of insertion*

The angle varies according to the anatomical region to be needled, the direction in which Qi sensation will be propagated and what is needed therapeutically.

There are three possible types of insertion: perpendicular, oblique and horizontal (Fig. 2.22).

*a. Perpendicular insertion.* The needle stands at an angle of 90° to the surface of the skin. This angle of entry is the one used throughout training and is appropriate for the majority of acupuncture points.

In perpendicular insertion the tip of the needle should always be pointed towards an imaginary central axis running through either the practice cushion, or the patient's trunk or limbs. This makes it easier to obtain Qi.

*b. Oblique insertion.* The needle stands at an angle of 45° to the surface of the skin. Those areas situated over important organs are usually needled in this way, for example Zhongfu LU 1 and Qimen LIV 14 on the chest. The tip of the needle is aimed towards the site of the disease to send Qi sensation in the desired direction more easily.

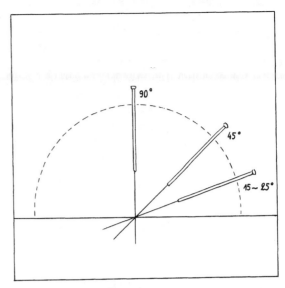

**Fig. 2.22** Angles of insertion.

*c. Horizontal insertion, also known as 'skimming the skin'.* The needle stands at an angle of 15° to the surface of the skin. This type of needling is used for points around the head, for example: Baihui Du 20, Shangxing Du 23.

### *Depth of insertion*

The depth of insertion varies according to the points needled. It must be increased or decreased according to the patient's age and physical constitution, the intensity of reaction, the level of the disease and the linking together of the points selected.

*a. Patient's age.* The depth of needling recommended by textbooks is suitable for adults. When needling children and the elderly, whose Blood and Qi is deficient, insertion should be less deep.

*b. Constitution.* Deeper needling can be used on big people with a strong constitution, whereas insertion should be less deep on thin patients with a weak constitution.

*c. Reaction to needling.* If the sensations of aching, numbness, distension or electric shock are very strong, or if these reactions occur very rapidly in nervous or timid patients, insertion should be less deep. Conversely needling should be deeper if reactions are slow to occur or not particularly strong.

*d. Level of the disease*. Chapter 50 of the *Su Wen* states that insertion should be superficial when the disease is on the surface, and that needling can be deeper when the disease is internal.

*e. Joining points*. Linking points together increases Qi sensation in the same way as varying the depth and/or length of insertion. It is accomplished by needling one point through to another. According to the way the needle is inserted needling can be:

- horizontal under the skin, e.g. Dicang ST 4 to Jiache ST 6,
- oblique, e.g. Hegu LI 4 to Laogong P 8,
- perpendicular, e.g. Neiguan P 6 to Waiguan TB 5.

*Examples of joining points:*

— Rebellious migraine:
   Sizhukong TB 23 to Shuaigu GB 8
— Paralysis of the upper eyelid:
   Zanshu Bl 2 to Yuyao (extra point)
— Deviation of the mouth:
   Quanliao SI 18 to Xiaguan ST 7
— Toothache in the upper jaw:
   Taiyang (extra point) to Xiaguan ST 7
— Elbow pain:
   Quchi LI 11 to Shaohao HT 3
— Arthritis of the shoulder:
   Tiaokou ST 38 to Chengshan BL 57
— Acute stomach pain:
   Juque Ren 14 to Zhongwan Ren 12
— Arterial hypertension:
Taichong LIV 3 to Yongquan KID 1.

## Correct sequence of needling

In general the order in which points are needled goes from top to bottom; in other words the points in the upper part of the body are needled first. When using bilateral treatments, a point on one side is needled, followed by the same point on the other side. If the condition of the disease requires starting on the lower part of the body, then the order of insertion should be from the bottom to the top.

In no case should points be needled here and there at random. If the needles are left in place, they should be withdrawn in the order of insertion.

## Practitioner's behaviour during treatment

*Su Wen*, Chapter 54:

The right hand should be very firm, as if restraining a tiger. The Shen should be free of all outside preoccupations, contemplating the patient calmly and brooking no distraction. The needle should go in straight, without veering off to one side.

*Biao Yu Fu*:

His hand is held as if restraining a tiger, he keeps his eyes from straying. The Shen should not be dispersed, but is concentrated as if waiting for someone important.

Thus the practitioner's hand is solid and firm, his grip is never tentative. The acupuncturist should focus his whole mind on the patient's body and his reaction to the needle. By observing the patient's face, his bearing, and his reaction to stimulation, and looking out for possible changes in facial colour, signs of stress or fear he can detect "needle shock" in time.

Finally, one of the keys to success in therapy is obtaining Qi, so before any treatment, and especially if it is the first session, the practitioner should give an explanation to the patient of any reactions that could arise from inserting the needle (aching, numbness, distension, heaviness or electric shock sensation). The patient should understand that all these sensations are normal and that they should be described to the acupuncturist as soon as they arise. The practitioner should also encourage the patient not to be frightened and not to move around.

In this way the recommendations of the *Ling Shu* (Ch. 1) can be respected: the acupuncturist should listen to the patient attentively and put his Shen into the needle.

## Complications following needling

### Blackout, syncope, convulsions, 'needle shock'

### Aetiology:

- First acupuncture treatment, patient anxious
- Oversensitive nature, weak constitution
- Overstimulation, inappropriate treatment.

### Symptoms:

*Mild cases:*

- Vertigo/dizziness, pallor, nausea

- Palpitations, uneasy feeling
- Cold sweat.

*Serious cases:*

- Face white and waxy, limbs shivering
- Pulse fine (Xi) and weak (Ruo)
- Sudden fainting.

### Prevention:

- If it is the patient's first ever acupuncture session, dispel his fears by explaining to him what he may feel from the needle.
- Use light, gentle manipulation on people with a weak constitution, the elderly, children, pregnant women and in cases of chronic illness.
- Avoid using acupuncture on people who are undernourished, exhausted or very anxious.
- Place the patient in a comfortable position.

**Treatment:** For practitioners who leave the needles in place (see below, Ch. 3):

- Take out all the needles immediately.
- Get the patient to lie down with his head low, loosen his clothes, give him a hot drink and leave him to rest.
- For loss of consciousness the classical treatment is to needle Yongquan KID 1, Renzhong Du 26 or Hegu LI 4, Shaochong HT 9, Baihui Du 20, Zusanli ST 36, or to put moxa on Baihui and Zusanli.

For those who do not leave the needles in place, as recommended in this book, the problem of taking them out does not arise.

Needling and manipulation of Suliao Du 25 (½–1 cun in depth) is advised, which will bring the patient round immediately. Never leave the needle in place.

### Pricking a vein

Puncture of a vein is painful and should not be confused by the patient with the arrival of Qi. The patient feels an unbearable burning sensation and is aware that the pain comes from the needle.

If pricking a vein has caused bleeding or a haematoma press the point firmly with the thumb for 1–3 minutes. Repeat if necessary and follow with a moxa stick over the general area to disperse the blood.

### Hitting a peripheral nerve

If the needle hits a nerve the pain is very intense. To retract the needle use moxa. Warm the area around the needle and gently pull it out.

Interpreting trauma to the nervous sheath as the arrival of Qi, then manipulating the needle in error may lead to neuritis.

### If the needle gets stuck

A needle is considered 'stuck' if it temporarily cannot be manipulated after insertion. It is impossible to rotate the needle, push it in deeper or take it out.

### Aetiology:

- Pain
- The skin and the tissues around the point have contracted strongly
- Rotating the needle in one direction only has entwined subcutaneous or muscular fibres around it
- The needle has been left in place for too long and the patient has changed position.

### Treatment:

- Use your fingers to tap or press on the place where the needle is stuck, or use moxa on the end of the needle.
- Put another needle into a point next to the place where the needle is stuck, or into the corresponding point on the other side.
- If there are fibres entwined around the needle, rotate it in the opposite direction before withdrawing it.
- Put the patient back in his original position.

### If the needle gets bent

The body of the needle gets bent or twisted into a zig-zag or hook inside the area needled. The needle is 'imprisoned' in the tissues and resists manipulation. The patient is in great pain.

### Causes:

- The manipulation was too forceful.
- Excessive muscular contraction: the patient was unable to bear the stimulation from the needle.

- The patient changed position.
- The tip of the needle encountered a hard surface.

### Prevention:

- Place the patient in a comfortable position; he should remain in that position.
- Manipulate the filiform needle smoothly. The force exerted by the fingers should be equal and regulated.
- If the needle is left in place be careful not to bend the handle when covering the patient with a blanket.

### Treatment:

- Do not withdraw the needle forcefully but keep turning and retracting it, following the direction of the curvature.

### If the needle snaps

If the needle snaps in situ the end will either be visible on the surface of the skin or out of sight.

### Causes:

- Poor quality needle
- Badly maintained needle
- Overused needle
- Too much force was used in the manipulation
- The muscular contraction was too strong.

### Prevention:

- Check the needle before insertion, particularly at the junction of handle and body.
- Perform the manipulations smoothly.
- Don't push the body of the needle all the way in.
- Don't change the patient's position.

### Treatment:

- If the broken end of the needle protrudes from the skin, instruct the patient not to move. With a pair of tweezers push the skin down around the needle to increase the length of the bit sticking out, then pull out the remainder.
- If the broken piece is not visible, the patient must not be moved lest the needle penetrate further, and surgical extraction should be carried out immediately.

### Pricking an internal organ or other important organic structure

Practically all of Chapter 52 of the *Su Wen* is devoted to listing the possible risks to the internal organs and other important organic structures from poorly mastered or badly aimed needling.

#### a. Lungs

Needling too deep in the depression inferior to the clavicle, on the back or on the anterior aspect of the chest could lead to traumatic pneumothorax.

### Symptoms:

- Pain
- Dyspnoea, oppression in the chest
- Cyanosis
- Profuse sweating
- Shock, even pulmonary collapse
- Lack of vesicular murmur on the affected side
- Occasionally there are no symptoms until much later.

### Prevention:

- Never needle deeper than 1 cun. Oblique or horizontal insertion is preferable.
- Never use lifting and thrusting (Ti Cha), only manipulations involving rotation.

### Treatment:

- Put the patient into a semi-upright position.
- If dyspnoea and other symptoms persist, seek emergency assistance.

#### b. Liver, spleen, kidneys

Puncturing one of these organs can lead to haemorrhaging with pain in the area of the affected organ combined with shock.

#### c. Gall bladder, stomach, intestines, bladder

Puncture of these organs can lead to peritonitis.

#### d. Spinal cord, medulla, nerve roots

- Badly applied needling at Yamen Du 15, Fengfu Du 16, Fengchi GB 20 can lead to a lesion of the medulla.

- Needling of the Hua Tuo Jia Ji point level with the first lumbar vertebra can lead to injury to the spinal cord.
- Injury to a peripheral nerve root can lead to neuritis.

## Contraindications for acupuncture

Contraindications for acupuncture are determined either by the condition of the patient or by the nature of the point.

### Contraindications relating to the condition of the patient

The following rules prohibiting needling are set out in the *Su Wen*, Chapter 52:

Needling should never be given to patients who are drunk, for their Qi has been routed, nor to those in a rage, for their Qi is ebbing, nor to those who are starving or those who have just eaten, nor to those with great thirst or those in great fear.

The *Ling Shu* clarifies these rules in Chapter 9:

A patient should never be treated just after sexual intercourse. Similarly he should not have intercourse immediately after the session. Acupuncture should never be given to a man who is drunk, and after the session the patient should not drink alcohol. People should not be needled after a fit of rage or great anger and should take care not to become angry after the session. A patient should not be needled if he is in a state of exhaustion and should never tire himself out after acupuncture.

The physician should not give acupuncture to someone who has just eaten a big meal and after the session the patient should not have too much to eat. Similarly a patient who is extremely hungry should not be needled or go too long without food after the session. Someone who is extremely thirsty should never be needled. Conversely, the patient should not go too long without drinking after the session. If the patient has had a bad fright he should have time to get over it before being needled. In the same way someone who has travelled a long way should not be needled immediately, but should be left to rest for as long as it takes to eat a meal [20 to 30 minutes]. If the patient has come a long way by foot he should also be left to rest, for as long as it takes to walk 10 Li [about 5 km].

In Chapter 61 the *Ling Shu* describes a contraindication relating to the nature of the disease:

Patients can suffer from five kinds of deficiency due to loss of Qi. If the patient has been ill for a long time, if his muscles are wasted and he is getting weaker and weaker this is generally due to his Qi becoming exhausted. Loss of Qi may also occur when the patient has lost a lot of blood and has been unable to replenish it. The third kind of loss of Qi occurs after incessant and profuse sweating has depleted the patient of fluids. The fourth kind follows severe uncontrolled diarrhoea, when the patient is very weak. The fifth kind concerns women in confinement who have lost a lot of blood and whose energy is therefore depleted. In these five conditions the physician should never use reducing techniques.

Chapter 61 of the *Ling Shu* also makes it clear that acupuncture should not be given in cases of 'contradictory' illness, where the pulse does not match the patient's symptoms:

In febrile diseases the patient's pulse should be full and broad. If it is small and calm then the disease is developing in an abnormal and "contradictory" way. After profuse sweating the pulse should be calm and small. If it is full and rapid then the disease is developing in a "contradictory" way. These two conditions form the first category of "contradictory" disease. In cases of severe diarrhoea the pulse should also be quiet. If it is big it corresponds to a second group of diseases developing in a "contradictory" way.

A third category of "contradictory" disease manifests itself when the patient's legs are paralysed and without sensation, and when after a long period in bed the muscles around his knees appear to putrefy. The patient is then feverish and his pulse is very weak.

The fourth type corresponds to a disease which has attacked the interior of the body and considerably weakened the patient. He is feverish, with a dull pale complexion and passes stools containing black blood. In this case the disease has taken a particularly grave turn.

If after a long and serious illness the patient is emaciated and weak, his pulse too should normally be weak. If however he has a strong pulse then he fits the fifth category of "contradictory" disease.

### Contraindications relating to the nature of the point

The following contraindications are given by Yang Ji Zhou in the *Zhen Jiu Da Cheng*:

Litany of forbidden points

| | | | | | |
|---|---|---|---|---|---|
| Naohu | Du 17 | Xinhui | Du 22 | Shenting | Du 24 |
| Yuzhen | BL 9 | Luoque | BL 8 | Chengling | GB 18 |
| Luxi | TB 19 | Jiaosun | TB 20 | Chengqi | ST 1 |
| Chengjin | BL 56 | Sanyangluo | TB 8 | Ruzhong | ST 17 |
| Shendao | Du 11 | Lingtai | Du 10 | Shanzhong | Ren 17 |
| Shuifen | Ren 9 | Shenque | Ren 8 | Huiyin | Ren 1 |
| Hengu | KI 11 | Qichong | ST 30 | Jimen | SP 11 |
| Shousanli | LI 10 | Qingling | HT 2 | | |

Hegu LI 4 and Sanyinjiao SP 6 should not be needled in pregnancy. Shimen Ren 5 should not be needled or treated with moxa on women as it can make them sterile.

Yunmen LU 2, Jiuwei Ren 15, Quepen ST 12 and Jianjing GB 21 can all give rise to syncope, which can be treated by needling Zusanli ST 36.

Thus the classics advise that points situated over the organs or important structures should not be needled.

Recent clinical experience shows that these prohibitions can be divided into three categories:

1. It is strictly forbidden to needle some points, for example: Rhuzhong ST 17, Shenque Ren 8.

2. Other points should be used with extreme caution, for example: points on the lower abdomen on pregnant women. If the pregnancy has reached three months or more, points on the lumbar or sacral region should not be used. The same applies to Hegu and Sanyinjiao, and other points which cause a strong reaction, to avoid risk of miscarriage. In cases of necessity these points can be needled but great care must be taken.

3. Some points may be used discerningly (depth of insertion, strength of reaction), for example: points near the organs, important structures and large blood vessels. In these cases superficial oblique insertion can be used.

# 3. Obtaining Qi (De Qi)

*Ling Shu*, Chapter 1:

The most important thing in acupuncture is the arrival of Qi.

*Su Wen*, Chapter 54:

Whether the Qi is far away or close at hand, the insertion superficial or deep, the aim is always to summon Qi.

*Su Wen*, Chapter 25:

When the Qi in the channel has arrived, the physician must take great care not to lose it.

Obtaining Qi (De Qi) results from inserting the needle into the selected point correctly, to the depth required. It is signalled by particular kinds of sensation felt by the patient and the practitioner.

For the patient, the arrival of Qi is distinguished by one of the following kinds of sensation: aching (Suan), numbness (Ma), distension (Zhang), heaviness (Zhong), tiredness (Kun), cold (Liang), warmth (Re), or electric shock (Chu Dian). These different sensations are usually felt around the needle but may move up or down the pathway of the channel, or diffuse outwards from the point.

For the practitioner, the arrival of Qi is distinguished by a gripping sensation around the needle deep inside the tissues, or a feeling of pressure underneath the needle pushing it upwards. The practitioner should notice this sensation a moment before the patient tells him about it. He may also feel a kind of pulling when manipulating the needle or notice muscular tremors around or some distance away from the point.

Obtaining Qi includes methods of stimulating Qi when it is slow to arrive and methods of moving Qi and preserving it once it has arrived.

## THEORY

### A. QI SENSATION

When Qi arrives at the needle, the sensation experienced by the patient can take various forms. Different types of 'Qi sensation' can develop in the course of the manipulation, passing through different levels of intensity ranging from slight to very intense, or even painful. The patient may also experience some of these in combination.

The different types of 'Qi sensation' felt by the patient and/or the practitioner are described below in increasing order of intensity.

#### Types of sensation

1. Itching.
2. Numbness.
3. Aching.
4. The three kinds of sensation above can change and develop into a sensation of swelling.
5. The patient can experience sensations of greater intensity: distension or heaviness comparable to the feeling of internal pressure produced by an intramuscular injection of a concentrate, or of liquid anaesthetic in dental surgery.
6. The sensation experienced may also be a mixture in varying degrees of the first five.

It is preferable to elicit all these sensations, either on their own or in combination, with the minimum possible pain.

7. This category relates to what is sometimes observed by the practitioner. The sensation consists of a feeling of constriction around the needle:

the practitioner senses that the tissues have closed up around it and have seized it with quite some force. It often accompanies one of sensation types 1–6 described above, which the patient may feel to a greater or lesser degree.

It is only when the practitioner has obtained the first sensations (nos. 1–6) on the patient, or noticed sensation type 7, that he can consider carrying out those manipulations which require that 'Qi must have been obtained beforehand'.

When the needle is gripped by Qi (sensation type 7), but the Qi contains Perverse energy, the sensation of constriction is powerful. The needle feels as if it is glued in place, often giving a sensation of suction towards the base. It is nevertheless possible to rotate the needle, but only with difficulty. In treatment this signifies a condition which should be followed by reducing techniques.

When the needle is held by True Qi (Zhen Qi), the sensation of constriction is slight, there is no sensation of suction towards the base and it is easier to rotate the needle. In treatment this type of sensation signifies a condition which should be followed by reinforcing techniques.

Care must be taken to differentiate properly between the gripping sensation caused by Qi and the sensation caused by muscular fibres which have become entwined around the needle. This is extremely constricting and painful for the patient, and can be confused with obtaining Qi. An experienced practitioner can easily recognise the difference in sensation (by observing the elasticity of the skin at the site of the constriction, the level of pain, etc.).

8. Icy cold sensation. This is generally only a fleeting sensation.

9. Sensation of warmth. This sensation does not last long and manifests itself as either a warm comfortable feeling spreading out from the needle, or a painful burning sensation.

10. Jerking or trembling of the muscles. For example, needling Hegu LI 4 causes a movement of the index finger.

11. Electric shock. Of all the needle sensations this is the most desirable. It is the pinnacle of the art of precise needling. It should be the practitioner's goal to obtain this sensation as often as possible every time he inserts a needle.

If the patient feels electric shock sensation strongly then the manipulation is reducing the energy. If he only feels it slightly then it is reinforcing. In both cases, however, there is an 'ideal sensation', which is felt along the pathway of the channel for a distance of 30 cm or more (this is sometimes felt throughout the channel pathway from points on the limbs, or by the internal organs when the back Shu points are needled). When the sensation radiates locally the manipulation can be said to be Balancing (Ping Bu Ping Xie). A sensation of internal pressure which grows and diffuses to cover an area the size of a large coin also constitutes Balancing (Ping Bu Ping Xie).

The pain caused by needling a nerve fibre should be distinguished from electric Qi sensation. For example, needling Zusanli ST 36 will propagate Qi sensation towards Jiexi ST 41, even as far as Neiting ST 44. This will travel much more slowly than the painful sensation generated by hitting a nerve. With practice the practitioner can recognise electric Qi sensation by the patient's reaction, which is never misleading, even before the patient tells him about it.

When electric Qi has been obtained it is better to withdraw the needle straight away without completing the manipulation.

### Observations on obtaining Qi

1. A study carried out on 1019 cases showed that Qi sensation was obtained (De Qi) on 90% of the patients. *It was also noticed that the degree of Qi sensation increases with the number of times a prescription is repeated over a course of treatment.* Moreover, although the sensation of obtaining Qi is subjective, it was possible to make objective observations on variations in electrical resistance and potential as well as changes in temperature.

2. When the illness is chronic or the patient is weak, Qi will not arrive at the needle quickly. When the energy is deficient the sensation around the needle is weak. The stronger the energy the stronger the sensation.

3. When Qi sensation differs from one side of the body to the other, the energy is manifestly out of balance. If after manipulation an identical sensation is restored to both sides (e.g. needling

Zusanli ST 36 on left and right sides), the patient's energy has been reharmonised.

4. Obtaining Qi is relatively easy on:

- the Ashi points when they are tender to the touch
- the Reunion points of the channels (e.g. Xuanshong GB 39 or Sanyinjiao SP 6)
- the points situated around the major joints (e.g. Yanglingquan GB 34, Shousanli LI 10 or Zusanli ST 36).

5. It is possible that after being needled the patient may feel a sensation for the rest of the day. This is a welcome phenomenon as it focuses the mind on the area treated, thus augmenting the effects of the therapy. In order to diminish the discomfort, however, the points needled should be massaged in the direction of the channel. A more agreeable and diffuse sensation is thus maintained in the area treated, keeping the patient's attention focused there for a while without recalling the sharp sensation of the needle.

## B. PROPAGATION OF QI SENSATION AND EFFECTIVENESS OF TREATMENT

Moving the Qi sensation towards the location of the disease is one of the keys to successful treatment with the filiform needle (Hao Zhen).

This condition was defined as early as 1295 in the *Zhen Jing Zhi Nan* which said 'If Qi arrives quickly the results come quickly; if the Qi arrives slowly, there are no results,' and has been corroborated by numerous experiments. In a report on one of these, carried out in 1964 by the Institute of Research into Chinese Medicine, Zheng Kui-san states:

A group of patients was treated for atrophy of the optic nerve by needling Fengchi GB 20. The effectiveness of treatment varied according to the level of Qi sensation propagated:

— 77% for those on whom sensation was propagated as far as the eye.

— 68% for those who had sensation reaching as far as the forehead.

— 42% for those who only felt a localised reaction.

Similarly, with patients with only one eye affected, Qi sensation was propagated in general as far as the eye on the healthy side. On the other hand, the sensation remained localised on the affected side.

When the disease is in both eyes and the patient feels a different sensation on each side, the results will generally be better on the side where the sensation is strongest.

If, however, the sensation is localised at the start of a course of treatment and gradually moves with time to the eye, the patient's vision will improve.

The result is therefore dependent on the rapidity with which Qi is obtained and its propagation towards the site of the disease. The speed with which the sensation is propagated has already been calculated in the *Jin Zhen Fu* as a function of the length of the channels and the number of respirations. This is currently estimated to be between 2 and 10 cm per second. Thus in one minute it is possible to reach the site of the disease or to move Qi throughout one channel.

In cases of paralysis or paraesthesia when the sensation does not move very far, another needle should be inserted into the spot where the sensation stops. This is what is called 'recapturing Qi' at the place where it has stopped. This enables the sensation to be propagated throughout the channel and to reach the site of the disease (strictly speaking this is now 'moving Qi'). For example, needling Jian Yu LI 15 should propagate sensation to the fingers. If the sensation stops at Quchi LI 11, Quchi must be needled so that the sensation can reach the fingers. However, the manipulation should not go on indefinitely. The quest for Qi sensation or the wish for this to reach as far as the 'site of the disease' does not mean that the patient's discomfort should be ignored.

## C. MOVING THE QI ACCORDING TO THE DISEASE

Moving Qi can be analysed in terms of the level of the disease and the nature of the disease.

### According to the level of the disease

It is important to take into account the level of the disease, i.e. whether it is external (Biao) or internal (Li), in order to determine where to obtain and move Qi.

Examples:

- In cases of Biao disease, and the skin, the disease is on the surface. The acupuncturist must wait for Qi at the level of heaven and make it move in the Couli[1] (see below, Ch. 4, 'Advancing and withdrawing').

• If the disease is in the muscles or the channels and collaterals (Jing Luo), or is half exterior (Biao) and half interior (Li), the acupuncturist should wait for Qi on the level of man and move Qi on the level of the channels and collaterals.

• If the disease is in the organs (Zang Fu), the bones or the marrow, and when there is pain, the acupuncturist should wait for Qi at the level of earth, and circulate it to rebalance the organs and stop the pain.

The *Zhen Jiu Da Cheng* says: 'In Cold or Hot disease it is appropriate to move Qi at the level of Heaven; in diseases of the Jing Luo, it is appropriate to move Qi at the level of Man; in cases of paraesthesia, numbness, and pains Qi should be moved at the level of Earth.'

### According to the nature of the disease

The practitioner needs to decide whether to use reinforcing (tonification) or reducing techniques. This depends on whether the disease is Empty (Deficient) or Full (Excess).
Examples:

— In a chronic disease, an Empty condition manifesting itself in shortness of breath, loose stools, and a weak soft pulse, Reinforcing methods should be used. The same applies when there is a sensation of emptiness during insertion, of emptiness under the point of the needle or a feeling of softness or emptiness as the needle is pulled back. Use shaking (Tan), winding up (Nian), thrusting (Ti) or pressing (An) until the presence of energy is felt, until the needle is gripped and there is a feeling of warmth propagating to fill the Emptiness.

— When the disease is recent, acute and a Full condition (Excess) or manifests itself in oppression of the chest, abdominal pains, constipation and a strong big pulse (Da) it is appropriate to use Reducing methods. The same applies when there is a sensation of tightness around the needle during insertion, if insertion feels bumpy, and if there is a feeling of great constriction deep inside, or as the needle is pulled back. Use lifting (Cha), shaking (Yao), following along (Xun) or pushing (She) to ease the sensation under the needle and generate a sensation of coolness to disperse the Fullness.

This is explained in the *Su Wen*, Chapter 54: 'When the needle fills an Emptiness it is warming and Fullness of Qi (True) manifests as Heat. When the needle drains a Fullness it is cooling and Emptiness of Qi (Perverse) manifests as Cold.'

---

## TECHNIQUES

---

The quality of the sensation (aching, tiredness, numbness, distension, warmth, coolness, electric shock, etc.), the distance and the direction in which Qi is propagated are closely linked to the needle manipulation, its duration, the precision with which the point is located and the state of the disease. The point should therefore be located correctly and the needle inserted to the appropriate depth. If the practitioner can detect no sign of obtaining Qi, if there is no sensation of Qi being propagated, or Qi is lost, then the following techniques should be used:

• waiting for Qi
• moving Qi
• maintaining Qi.

### WAITING FOR QI (Hou Qi)

'Waiting for Qi' means leaving the needle in place for a few seconds after insertion, without any manipulation.

If there is no sign of Qi then lifting and thrusting or rotation techniques can be used to make Qi arrive. However, it is better to use methods aimed at 'stimulating Qi'.

---

[1] Couli: 'designates the texture, the grain of the skin, the muscles as well as the connective tissue joining the muscles to the skin. It can be divided into Cou of the skin, Cou of the muscles, unrefined Li, refined Li, small Li, Li of the Heaters. It is the place where the body fluids penetrate, the door of communication between Qi and Blood, the cavity able to resist attack by External Evils' *Jiangming Zhongyi Cidian* (p. 992). Here Couli denotes the space between the skin and muscles.

### 1. Probing for Qi (Sou)

This technique is used when the needle has penetrated quite far but Qi has not yet been obtained. In this case, the needle should be withdrawn to just beneath the epidermis, pointed in a different direction and pushed back in. If Qi is still not obtained, the process is continued by lifting the needle and pushing it back in a few times. The needle is pointed forwards, backwards, to the left and to the right whilst 'probing' for Qi, until it arrives.

### 2. Massaging the channel pathway (Xun An)

If Qi has not arrived after insertion, the channel pathway of the point needled or the area around the point is massaged or tapped lightly (Figs. 3.1–3.3). This technique may also be used to resolve cases of 'stuck needle'.

### 3. Pushing (She)

Bunch the thumb, index and third finger of your right hand together. Use your fingertips to push down firmly at intervals on the area around the point (Fig. 3.4). This technique is also used to resolve 'stuck needle'.

### 4. Flicking (Tan Zhen)

'Tan' means flicking the handle of the needle to

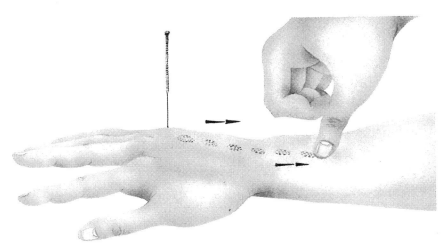

**Fig. 3.1** Massaging the channel pathway with the thumb to summon Qi.

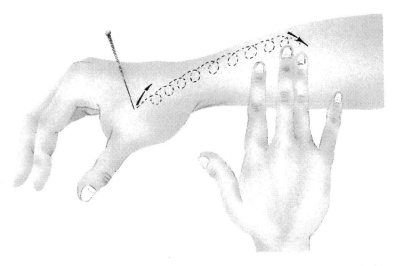

**Fig. 3.2** Massaging the channel pathway with the third finger to summon Qi.

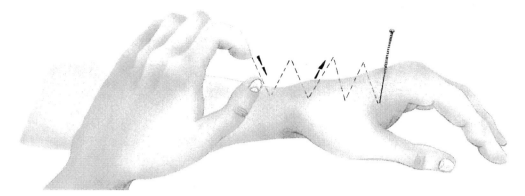

**Fig. 3.3** Tapping the channel pathway with the index finger to summon Qi.

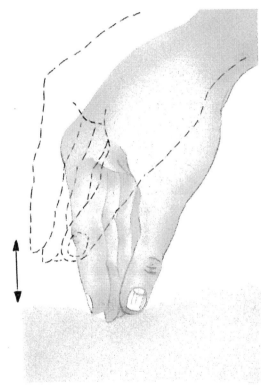

**Fig. 3.4** Pushing down at intervals around the point to summon Qi.

make Qi come and to elicit a sensation of gripping deep inside (Fig. 3.5).

'Zhen' means making a half fist with the third or index finger extended. The finger flicks the handle of the needle, making it shake. This stimulates the Qi of the channel and accelerates and increases Qi sensation.

### 5. *Bird pecking* (Que Zhuo)

This technique strongly increases Qi sensation. It is accomplished by a lifting and thrusting movement of small amplitude but great rapidity.

### 6. *Vibrating* (Chan)

This entails a 'lifting and thrusting' movement. The right hand vibrates up and down extremely rapidly but with tiny amplitude. This sensation is similar to that made by an electrical stimulator. The technique is extremely difficult to master and learning it is made easier by familiarity with and practice of Qi Gong exercise IV (see Ch. 10).

### 7. *Relocating the needle* (Yi Wei)

If the point has not been located properly, or the needle is correctly situated but angled wrongly, it should be relocated or reoriented before proceeding with manipulations to stimulate Qi. This will generally summon Qi straight away.

If the patient is paralysed in one or more limbs, or if needle sensation is very slow to come, Qi can be stimulated by the methods described above. However, if Qi still does not arrive, then more complex techniques should be used, for example 'Green tortoise seeks the point' (see Ch. 5). The needle is then left in place while the acupuncturist awaits the arrival of Qi.

## MOVING QI (Xing Qi)

When Qi has been obtained the practitioner may

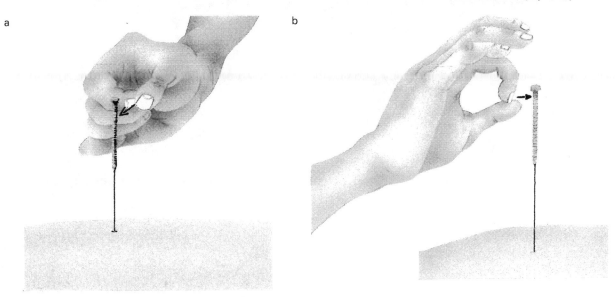

**Fig. 3.5a, b** Flicking to summon Qi.

use 'lifting and thrusting' (Ti Cha), 'rotation' (Cuo Nian), 'blocking' (Guan Bi), etc. These techniques are intended to increase needle sensation or to propagate it to an area further away.

### 1. Lifting and Thrusting (Ti Cha)

'Lifting' (Ti) means withdrawing the needle as far as the surface (Fig. 3.6). 'Thrusting' (Cha) means inserting the needle deeply (Fig. 3.7).

To make Qi move, 'Lifting and Thrusting' techniques are generally performed over a distance of 1 fen from the tip of the needle. This propagates Qi. There are, however, several variations of Ti Cha, each type applied according to the condition of the disease: light or strong, and rapid or slow. This technique can also be used to make Qi arrive.

### 2. Rotation (Cuo Nian)

'Cuo' means turning strongly, making the needle describe a large angle of rotation, generally more than 180°. 'Nian' means turning gently, with a very small angle of rotation, generally less than 45°. The rotation of the needle is always in one direction only, as if winding up a thread.

In clinical practice rotating the needle (Cuo Nian) after Qi has been obtained causes the sensation to spread. When using this technique the

needle should not be rotated too hard or too rapidly or it will get caught up in the fibres of the subcutaneous or muscular tissue and cause pain.

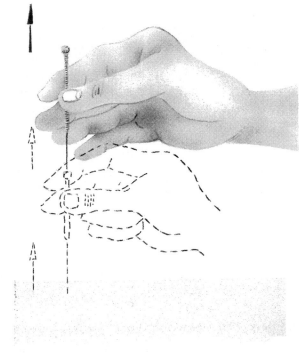

**Fig. 3.6** Ti: lifting the needle to the surface.

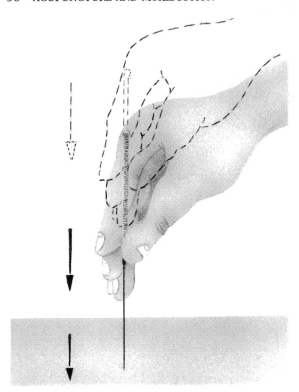

Fig. 3.7   Cha: thrusting the needle in deep.

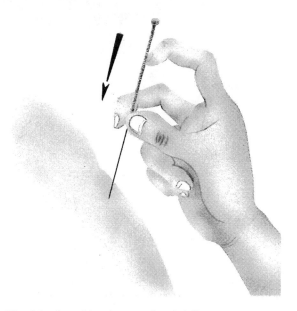

**Fig. 3.8**   Scratching downwards to reinforce.

### 3. *Swinging and Scratching* (Bo Gua)

'Bo': when Qi has arrived at the needle, the handle is held between the thumb and index finger of the right hand and swung like a pendulum. The swing travels through 45° from left to right and should be as slow as possible so the sensation spreads. This technique is also used to disperse knots and swellings.

'Gua': when Qi has arrived at the needle, the handle is either scratched upwards or downwards with the nail of the thumb or index finger of the right hand. This helps increase the sensation. Generally, however, scratching downwards is used to reinforce (Fig. 3.8), and scratching upwards is used to reduce (Fig. 3.9).

### 4. *Cranking and Shaking* (Pan Yao)

'Pan' means pushing the needle down as far as the level of earth (the point's maximum depth, or 'between the muscles and the bone'). After Qi is obtained the needle is withdrawn up as far as the level of man (the point's median depth or 'in the

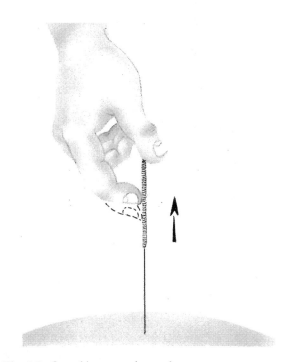

**Fig. 3.9**   Scratching upwards to reduce.

muscle') or the level of heaven ('under the skin'). The needle is inclined at 45° to the plane of the skin and turned round slowly, as if cranking a millstone (Fig. 3.10). Generally three revolutions

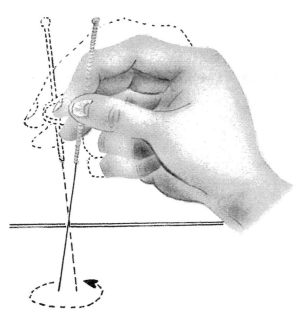

**Fig. 3.10**   Pan: lean the needle over and turn it slowly.

are enough. This technique helps to increase Qi sensation.

'Yao': when Qi has been obtained, the needle is swung from left to right through an angle of about 90°, like shaking a hand bell (Fig. 3.11). Generally three times are enough, allowing the hole made by the needle to broaden. 'Yao' technique is designed to spread the sensation further and creates emptiness under the needle. It is primarily a reducing technique.

Pan Yao should never be hurried or excessively rapid, or the muscles will seize up and immobilise the needle, causing swelling and pain and injuring the True Qi (Zhen Qi).

### 5. *Blocking* (Guan Bi)

After Qi has been obtained, use the thumb and index finger of the left hand to press on and block the area opposite the place towards which Qi should be propagated. Pressure is applied to the area where Qi is in abundance. The aim of this technique is to control and target the direction in which Qi is propagated.

If the sensation is intended to go upwards, the fingers of the left hand are placed beneath the point and exert a continuous upwards pressure. If the sensation is intended to go downwards, the

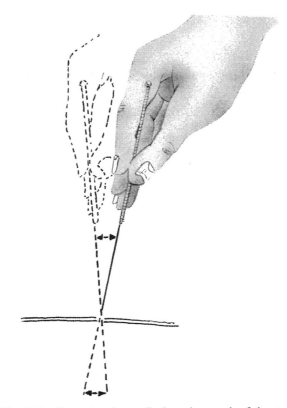

**Fig. 3.11**   Yao: swing the needle through an angle of about 90°.

fingers of the left hand are placed above the point and exert pressure downwards. Both hands work synergistically, pressing and directing together. In this way sensation can successfully be propagated to the site of the disease.

The action of the left hand is very important. It should not use too much pressure, as this could cause a blockage in the channel, or even move Qi in the wrong direction.

If the sensation type is numbness (Type 2), the left hand should press more firmly, whereas a lighter touch is required for swelling or distension (Types 4 and 5).

### 6. *Flying Away and Bending* (Fei Tui)

Flying Away (Fei) is similar to 'Nian', but the needle is only rotated once (Nian) then the thumb and index finger release the handle of the needle like a bird opening its wings to fly away (Fig. 3.12). The needle is rotated once, then the

a                                          b

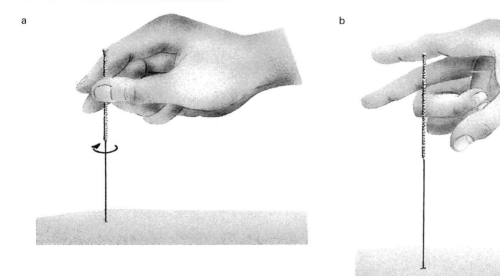

**Fig. 3.12a, b** Flying away. **a** Stage 1. **b** Stage 2.

handle is released once but in such a way that the needle is not made to rotate further.

'Tui' (Bending) is similar to 'Nian', but in 'Tui' the thumb and the index finger bend the handle of the needle forwards. In this case, too, the needle does not rotate.

These two methods enable needle sensation to be propagated to an area further away and prolong its duration.

'Fei' is also used to reinforce and reduce, while 'Tui' can be used to maintain Qi.

*Observations:*

1. Propagation of Qi sensation can be stopped in its flow by firm pressure or sufficiently low temperatures.

2. If the sensation stops near a major joint then stronger techniques should be used such as: 'Green dragon swings his tail', 'White tiger shakes his head', 'Green tortoise seeks the point' (see Ch. 5).

## C. MAINTAINING QI (Shou Qi)

If the patient feels Qi sensation after techniques to obtain and move Qi have been used, the sensation must be maintained. Both the *Ling Shu* and the *Su Wen* advise this: 'The good physician must know

how to maintain Qi' (*Ling Shu*, Ch. 3), 'When Qi has arrived, it is important to know how to maintain it' (*Su Wen*, Ch. 25).

To do this the techniques of 'Tui Nu' or 'Ban Dian' should be used.

*1. Cocking the crossbow* (Tui Nu)

The tip of the needle is leaned into the area of Qi sensation. The handle is held firmly between the right thumb, index and third fingers, then bent back as if cocking a crossbow, to stop the tip of the needle from losing contact with the area of Qi sensation. The needle is held for a few seconds to conserve and maintain the sensation.

*2. Moving the cushion* (Ban Dian)

'Ban' (moving): when Qi has been obtained and the patient has the appropriate sensation, the needle is held between thumb and index finger of the right hand. With index finger lower down on the handle than thumb, the needle is curved with the combined pressure of both fingers.

'Dian' (acting as a cushion): the right index finger moves down along the handle and acts as a cushion between the thumb and the skin. This blocks the area where there is sensation. Next the index finger moves back up and it is the

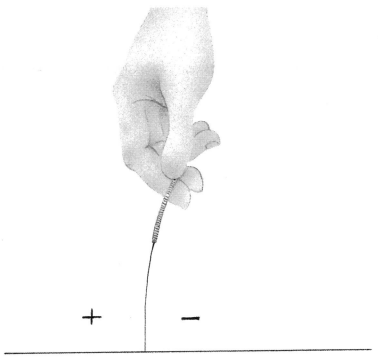

**Fig. 3.13**  Moving the cushion: the area reinforced is on the convex side of the needle, the area reduced on the concave side.

thumb's turn to act as a cushion, and so on. As with 'Ban', alternating the finger acting as the cushion, combined with pressure, increases the sensation.

This technique may be used to reinforce or to reduce. The part which is reinforced is on the convex side of the needle, the part reduced is on the concave side (Fig. 3.13).

# 4. Reinforcing, reducing and balancing

*Ling Shu*, Chapter 3:

A good physician will wait for the arrival of Qi. Only then will he practise reinforcing and reducing techniques to rebalance the patient's energy.

*Su Wen*, Chapter 25:

When the physician needles something which is empty, he must wait until it grows in strength. When he needles something which is full, he must wait until it grows weaker.

The 73rd difficulty in the *Nan Ching* explains that every needle manipulation can be used either to reinforce (Bu) or to reduce (Xie). These methods should be used discerningly, reinforcing in cases of deficiency of True Qi, and reducing in cases of fullness of Perverse Qi.

There are numerous methods of reinforcing and reducing:

## 1. Slow and Fast (Xu Ji )

The technique of inserting or withdrawing the needle rapidly or slowly determines whether the effect is reinforcing or reducing. The *Su Wen* (Ch. 54) says: 'To reinforce: slowness followed by rapidity . . . to reduce: rapidity followed by slowness'. The *Ling Shu* (Ch. 3) says: 'When the physician inserts the needle into a point slowly and withdraws it quickly it has a reinforcing effect. Conversely, the effect is reducing when the needle is inserted rapidly and withdrawn slowly'.

To reinforce, insert the needle slowly to the required depth and withdraw it rapidly to just below the skin, waiting for a second before taking it out. The aim is to make the Yang Qi penetrate into the interior.

To reduce, insert the needle rapidly and push it to the required depth in one movement, then withdraw it slowly little by little. The aim is to bring out the Perverse Qi from the interior to the surface.

**NB:** Although the above method is currently recognised as the best it is worth bearing in mind that time-honoured sources occasionally make contradictory assertions about the speed of needle insertion and withdrawal. Contradictions can even be found in the same work.

## 2. Lifting and Thrusting (Ti Cha)

The *Nei Jing* says: 'Lifting the needle is reducing, thrusting the needle in is reinforcing'.

Lifting and thrusting refers to the upward or downward movement of the needle when it has penetrated the skin. With this technique it is the force used to raise or lower the needle which determines whether the effect is reinforcing or reducing.

To reinforce, the needle is thrust forcefully from the surface to the interior, and pulled back gently. The aim is to use the strength with which the needle is dispatched to make the Yang Qi penetrate.

To reduce, the needle is withdrawn forcefully from the interior to the surface and thrust in gently. The aim is to draw the perverse energy to the exterior.

## 3. Advancing and Withdrawing (Jin Tui)

This technique divides the depth of the point into three equal stages: the superficial level is called the 'level of heaven', the middle level is called 'man', and the deep level 'earth'.

Reinforce by advancing the needle in three steps

(heaven–man–earth), and withdrawing it in one movement. This is what is called '3 advances, 1 withdrawal'.

Reduce by thrusting the needle straight to the level of earth and then withdrawing it in three stages. This is what is called '1 advance, 3 withdrawals' (Fig. 4.1).

**NB:** These three techniques are often used together to reinforce True Qi (Zhen Qi) or reduce Perverse Qi. They treat all Empty or Full conditions of Hot and Cold.

### 4. *Going against and Following* (Ying Sui)

The *Ling Shu* (Ch. 1) says, 'If the physician needles in the direction of the flow of the channel, it will reinforce the energy: this is tonification. If he needles against the flow it will weaken the energy: this is dispersing.' and (Ch. 9), 'When the physician reinforces he needles in the direction of the channel, when he reduces he needles against the flow of the channel'. In the first case the needle follows the Qi to support it, in the second it goes against the Qi to diminish it.

To reinforce, the needle is inserted obliquely in the direction of the flow of the channel. If the needle has been inserted perpendicularly, it should be withdrawn to just beneath the skin and reinserted obliquely, the tip pointing in the direction of the channel. If several points on the same channel are to be used, they should be needled consecutively following the flow of the channel.

To reduce, the needle should be inserted obliquely in the opposite direction to the flow of Qi in the channel. If the needle has been inserted vertically, it should be withdrawn to just under the skin, the tip pointed against the flow of Qi in the channel and then reinserted. If several points on the same channel are to be used, they should be needled consecutively in the opposite direction of the flow of the channel.

### 5. *Rotation* (Nian Zhuan)

'Nian' means rolling the needle between the fingers through a very small angle of rotation, generally 45–90°.

'Zhuan' means rolling the needle between the fingers through a very large angle of rotation, generally more than 180°.

To reinforce, the rotation should be abrupt, moving anti-clockwise through 45–90°. Pull your thumb towards you then put it back in position.

To reduce, rotate the needle clockwise through 180–360°. Extend the thumb away from you then put it back in position. The movement should be more fluid than for reinforcing (Fig. 4.2).

The direction of rotation recommended here,

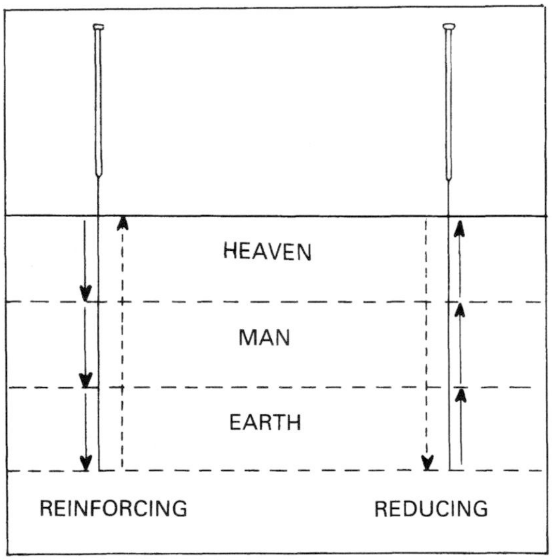

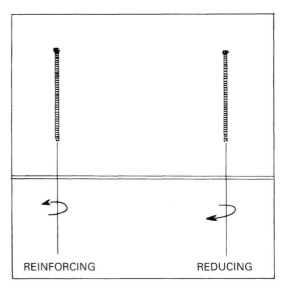

**Fig. 4.1** The 3 levels.

HEAVEN

MAN

EARTH

REINFORCING     REDUCING

**Fig. 4.2** Rotating the needle.

REINFORCING     REDUCING

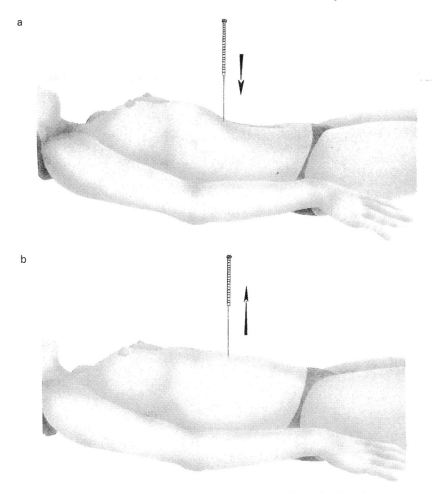

**Fig. 4.3a, b** Reinforcing. **a** Thrust the needle in as the patient breathes out. **b** Withdraw the needle as the patient breathes in.

although appearing to contradict what is taught by many schools, is based on interpretation of the oldest teachings of Chinese medicine, the *Luo Shu* and the *He Tu*.[1] In any case, there are many theories about direction of needle rotation. Yang Ji Zhou, for example, has developed a theory, based on the idea of 'going against and following' which says:

for the three arm Yang and the three leg Yin channels:
— reinforce by pulling your thumb towards you,
— reduce by extending your thumb away from you,
for the three leg Yang and the three arm Yin channels:

— reinforce by extending your thumb away from you,
— reduce by pulling your thumb towards you.

*Although it seems to us that the direction of rotation is not as important as the size of rotation, we have kept the information derived from the* He Tu *and the* Luo Shu. *In complex manipulations which combine lifting and thrusting movements with rotation, however, the techniques will be easier to practise if the methods we propose are followed.*

### 6. Breathing (Hu Xi)

*Su Wen* (Ch. 62):

To reinforce Emptiness, the needle is inserted as the patient breathes out. As soon as Fullness is established the needle is withdrawn rapidly as the patient breathes in.

---

The *He Tu*: a diagram, so tradition has it, brought to the emperor Fu Xi by a dragon-horse from the river. The *Luo Shu*: a diagram symbolising the world, brought to Yu the Great by a tortoise from the River Luo showing the numbers 1–9 arranged in a magic square.

a

b

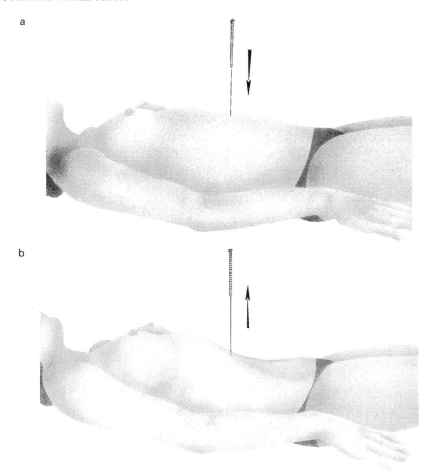

**Fig. 4.4a, b** Reducing. **a** Thrust the needle in as the patient breathes in. **b** Withdraw the needle as the patient breathes out.

To reduce Fullness, the needle is inserted where the Qi is in excess; through the opening thus presented the Qi accompanies the needle as the patient breathes out.

Reinforcing and reducing depend therefore on whether the needle is inserted or withdrawn as the patient breathes in or out. This technique is derived from the fundamental principles of 'going against and following'.

To reinforce, insert the needle as the patient breathes out (Fig. 4.3a) and withdraw it as he breathes in (Fig. 4.3b). To reduce, insert the needle as the patient breathes in (Fig. 4.4a) and withdraw it as he breathes out (Fig. 4.4b).

You reinforce when the needle follows the direction of the Qi (Shun Qi), and reduce when the needle goes against the normal direction of the Qi (Ni Qi).

Qi penetrates into the chest when the patient breathes in. If the needle is inserted at this moment, it will be in opposition to the Qi. When the patient breathes out, Qi leaves the chest and the abdominal wall becomes empty and subsides. If the needle is withdrawn at this moment the Qi follows the exit of the needle and thus excess is eliminated.

When the patient breathes out, Qi goes out, the abdomen is empty and Qi is weak. Inserting the needle at this moment reinforces True Qi (Zhen Qi) and fills Emptiness. The needle is in harmony with the movement of Qi. If the needle is withdrawn when the patient breathes in, the abdomen is full and the Qi is plentiful. True Qi is maintained, not dispersed, thus reinforcing the energy.

**NB:** There are two other alternative methods of breathing to reinforce or reduce:

1. If after needle insertion and arrival of Qi sensation, the needle is rotated:
- to reinforce, stop rotating the needle when the patient breathes in,
- to reduce, stop rotating the needle when the patient breathes out.

2. When manipulating the needle, it is preferable:
- to breathe in through the nose and breathe out through the mouth when reinforcing,
- to breathe in through the mouth and breathe out through the nose when reducing.

## 7. Opening and Closing (Kai He)

*Su Wen* (Ch. 54):

When reducing excessive Perverse Qi (Xie) which is victorious, the point should not be massaged when the needle has been taken out.

*Su Wen* (Ch. 62):

The hole should not close before the disease has found its way out, so the way is prepared by moving the needle to enlarge the hole.
As soon as the energy has been reinforced, the needle is withdrawn and the hole is closed.

To reinforce, the tip of the needle is brought to just beneath the skin in one brisk movement and held there for a fraction of a second. Pull the needle out quickly and massage the point.

To reduce, the needle is withdrawn slowly. It is lifted slowly and smoothly until it is out, swung from side to side, or moved in a spiral to enlarge the mouth of the hole. Once the needle is out, the point should not be touched.

Before withdrawing the needle make sure it is not caught up in any subcutaneous or muscular fibres by giving it a small rotation to disengage it.

## 8. Nine and Six (Jiu Liu)

This technique is based on the theory of the *I Ching*, and associates Yin with even numbers, and Yang with odd numbers. Broadly speaking, the odd number 9, which is Yang, is used to reinforce, and the even number 6, which is Yin, is used to reduce. This technique is used in conjunction with Rotation (Nian Zhuan) or with Lifting and Thrusting (Ti Cha).

To reinforce, the needle should be thrust in forcefully and lifted gently 9 times, or the needle should be rotated by pulling your thumb towards you 9 times. If the result is not satisfactory, the operation should be repeated in multiples of 9 ($3 \times 9 = 27$ times).

To reduce, the needle should be thrust in gently and withdrawn strongly 6 times, or rotated by extending your thumb away from you 6 times. If the perverse energy is very strong and has not been successfully reduced, the operation should be repeated in multiples of 6 ($2 \times 6 = 12$ times).

## 9. Retaining the needle (Liu Zhen)

The question of whether to retain the needle or withdraw it immediately after manipulation has always been controversial. In the West most acupuncturists are in favour of leaving the needle in place; it should be pointed out, however, that contrary to the teachings of the classics they use very little manipulation of the needle, if at all. In either case, *obtaining Qi is a must.*

*Ling Shu* (Ch. 1):

Once Qi has arrived there is no further need to retain the needle in the patient's body as the aim of the manipulation has now been achieved.

*Ling Shu* (Ch. 3):

A good physician withdraws the needle as soon as Qi arrives.

Whilst recognising that retaining the needle without any manipulation will increase and prolong its effect, we maintain that *after Qi has been obtained and proper manipulation the needle may be withdrawn immediately.*

Furthermore, several ancient texts state that removing the needle after obtaining Qi is reinforcing, and that leaving the needle until Qi has dispersed is reducing. Indeed, if the needle is left in place too long, the patient may complain of fatigue at the end of the session or for the next few days.

In clinical practice it is usually the condition of the disease which determines the treatment.

Examples:

— The needles are not left in place in the following cases:
- acute conditions needing emergency treatment (syncope, shock, collapse),

- children's diseases,
- diseases where it is established practice to withdraw the needles after obtaining Qi and correct manipulation.

— The needles may be retained after manipulation:

- in Cold diseases, cramps, spasms and violent pains,
- in nervous conditions, when the aim is sedative.

## NB

1. For teaching purposes the 9 techniques of reinforcing and reducing have been described separately. In practice, however, these differing manipulations are used in combination to form the complex needle manipulations studied in the next chapter.

2. *If the reinforcing technique is successful there will be a feeling of warmth or constriction of the fibres under the needle. If the reducing technique is successful there will be an emptiness under the needle as if it were standing in cream cheese or custard (soya cheese or tofu for the Chinese).*

## 10. Balancing: Reinforcing and Reducing equally (Ping Bu Ping Xie)

After insertion, Lifting and Thrusting (Ti Cha) and/or Rotation (Nian Zhuan) techniques are used. The rotation should be of medium amplitude, and in Lifting and Thrusting the same degree of force should be used for both downward and upward movements of the needle. When Qi arrives the needle should be withdrawn.

This technique is used primarily in cases where signs of Emptiness or Fullness are not very obvious, or in certain conditions manifesting both Emptiness and Fullness at the same time. It is also suitable for patients with a weak constitution who have been affected by a Full condition.

Certain complex needle manipulations, to be studied in the next chapter, are considered to be 'Reinforcing and Reducing Equally', for example:

— 'Yin hidden in Yang' or 'Hiding Yin in Yang',

— 'Yang hidden in Yin' or 'Hiding Yang in Yin',
— 'Dragon and tiger come to blows'.

This chapter ends with two reinforcing and reducing techniques which cannot be strictly classified as needle manipulations, but have often been described in this context in the classics. These are reinforcing and reducing according to the circulation of Qi in the channels and the Mother-Son technique.

### Reinforcing and Reducing according to the circulation of Qi in the channels (Na Zhi)

*Su Wen* (Ch. 54):

The timing (of reinforcing and reducing) should be in harmony with the movements of Qi in the channels.

*Ling Shu* (Ch. 75):

To treat Fullness, stimulate when the circulation of Qi has come to the channel. To treat Emptiness, stimulate when the circulation of Qi has left the channel.

Qi and Blood circulate in the channels through the action of Zhong Qi, ebbing and flowing according to the time of day, although Qi in the channel is also dependent on the condition of the organ (Zang or Fu) to which it belongs. Consequently, to reduce, the needle is inserted at the time of day when the Qi is at its strongest, 'going against' to eliminate excess: to reinforce, the needle is inserted when the Qi is weak, 'following' to treat deficiency.

### Mother-Son (Mu Zi)

This technique is used solely on the Shu points below the elbow and below the knee (known as the Su antique points) which are related to the Five Phases (Wu Xing) and the organs (Zang Fu).

In accordance with the cycles of controlling and promotion, the rule is to reinforce the Mother point (Mu) in Empty conditions (Xu), and reduce the Son point (Zi) in Full (Shi) conditions.

# 5. Filiform needle techniques

This chapter is crucial to the understanding of filiform needle manipulation. To make the best use of the information presented here the student should master both components, vertical and horizontal, of perpendicular insertion on the cushion, and assimilate the reinforcing and reducing techniques explained in the previous chapter.

The 16 techniques selected are the classical manipulations or their variations described in various key texts:

- *Zhen Jing Zhi Nan,*
- *Zhen Jiu Ju Yin,*
- *Zhen Jiu Wen Hui,*
- *Shen Ying Jing,*
- *Zhen Jiu Da Cheng.*

All of these manipulations, from the simplest to the most complex, are the result of using basic techniques in combination. They are difficult to classify, as the techniques of reinforcing, reducing and balancing are often the same as those designed to obtain or move Qi.

In this book, the techniques have been classified according to the level of skill involved in the manipulation, and arranged progressively from the simplest to the most difficult. The student should proceed methodically from one technique to the next, mastering each one in turn, so that it can be performed equally well vertically on top of the cushion and horizontally on the sides.

Practising on the cushion does not incorporate two basic concepts which are important in clinical practice.

— Before each and every manipulation, Qi must be obtained. Most reinforcing techniques can also be used to obtain Qi however, and can therefore be continued in the normal way when Qi arrives, unless the sensation obtained is electric Qi. In such cases withdraw the needle straight away and massage the point.

— Reinforcing is often accompanied by sensations of warmth whereas reducing is accompanied by sensations of coolness. The proportion of patients who feel warmth varies from 60–90% depending on the method used. Cool or cold sensation is much more difficult to obtain than warm sensation. It should also be noted that when the terms 'dragon' or 'tortoise' are applied to a manipulation in Chinese medicine, they denote that the technique is reinforcing, while the terms 'tiger' and 'phoenix' denote that the technique is reducing.

The techniques in this chapter are based on two key elements:

*1. The position of the right hand when holding the needle*

The success of the manipulation depends on this position. This is sufficiently important to warrant an entire section of this chapter. It should be understood that holding the needle correctly is an integral part and the starting point of each of the 16 techniques described.

*2. Opposition between active and passive movements*

Mastery of the manipulation depends on proper execution of these two movements, both complementary and opposed at one and the same time. This is demonstrated by the first two techniques below.

## HAND POSITIONS

### *Starting position*

Place the cushion in front of you, directly opposite the right axillary line of the body. With the left hand in tiger claw, very slowly insert a filiform needle perpendicularly to a suitable depth (1.2 cm).

### *Holding the needle*

Check that the needle has been inserted exactly at right angles to the surface of the cushion. Place the medial (the ringfinger side) edge of the nail of your right third finger on the cushion. The pad of the finger should be opposite the needle and perpendicular to the plane of your left index finger. *This movement requires that the hand should rotate to the right, bringing the first metacarpal of the right hand into a straight line drawn from the radial edge of the forearm.*

Next, flex the proximal interphalangeal joint of your third finger (PIP), keeping the distal interphalangeal joint (DIP) extended.

Hold your right little finger out, pointing in the air, with your right elbow close to your body and your shoulders down.

Keep your wrist turned slightly to the right to keep the first metacarpal in line with the radial edge of the forearm.

Finally, bring the centre of the pads of your right thumb and index finger towards each other to form an open angle around the needle and grasp it gently at the root.

This is the correct way to hold the needle (see Figs. 5.1–5.3).

## A. SIMPLE MANIPULATIONS

### 1. REINFORCING BY LIFTING AND THRUSTING (Ti Cha)

In this technique the *Reinforcing* elements of slow and fast (xu ji), lifting and thrusting (ti cha), and opening and closing (kai he) are used in combination in a simple manipulation.

### *Method*

Take hold of the needle and give it a short lifting and thrusting movement of around 1–2 mm, following the principle of the ancient texts: 'Thrust forcefully, lift gently'.

*The active movement of 'thrusting forcefully' is*

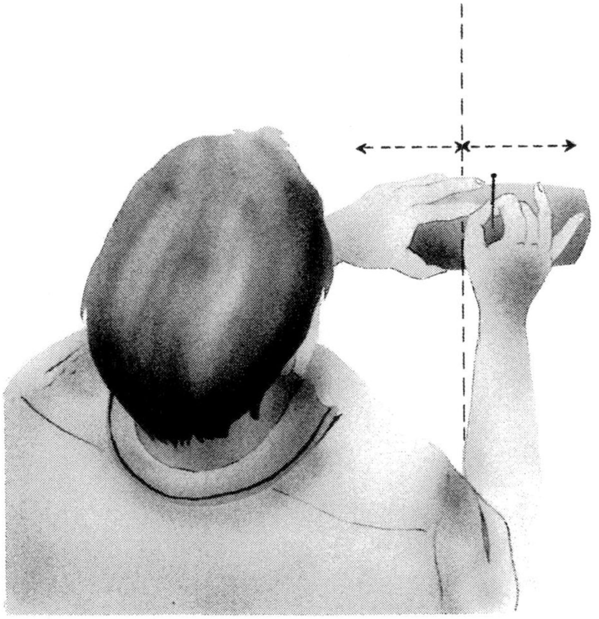

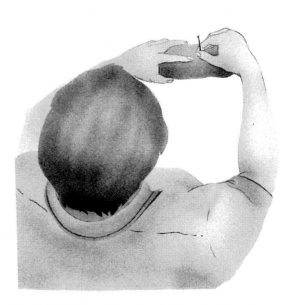

**Fig. 5.1**   Holding the needle: right hand positioned correctly on the cushion.

**Fig. 5.2**   Holding the needle: right hand positioned incorrectly on the cushion.

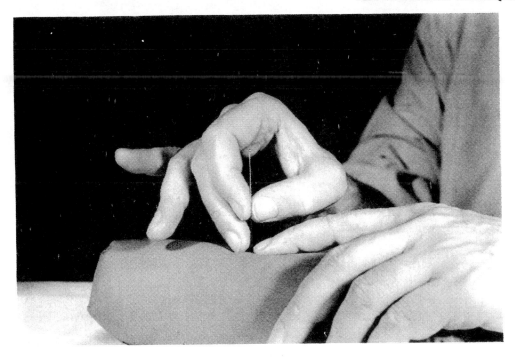

**Fig. 5.3** Holding the needle.

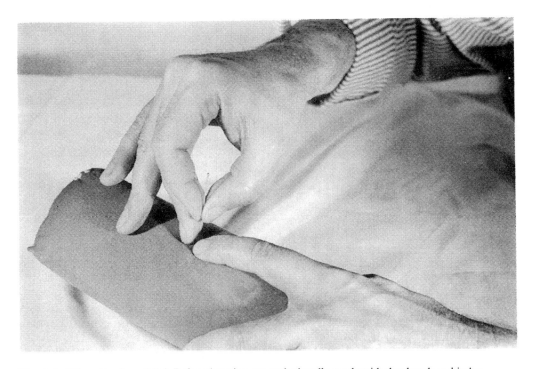

**Fig. 5.4** 'Thrusting forcefully'. Before thrusting, grasp the handle gently with the thumb and index finger, so the fingers form a circle.

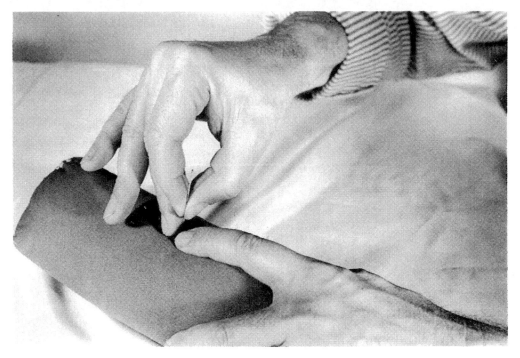

**Fig. 5.5** 'Thrusting forcefully'. As the needle is pushed in, the pincer closes in on itself, so the space between the fingers becomes more narrow.

accomplished through the movement of the thumb and index finger. These two digits form a pincer which extends forwards as they contract. It is this extension alone which causes the needle to penetrate, but the needle is withdrawn through the release of the contraction.

During the course of the movement a bulge should appear at the junction of the 1st and 2nd metacarpals, indicating that the muscle is in contraction and the manipulation is being performed correctly (Figs 5.4, 5.5).

Without hurrying, join the downward and upward movements of the needle together in one continuous, even and harmonious sequence for the duration of the treatment, usually 10–15 seconds.

Withdraw the needle swiftly and massage the point.

## 2. REDUCING BY LIFTING AND THRUSTING (Ti Cha)

In this technique the *Reducing* elements of slow and fast (xu ji), lifting and thrusting (ti cha), and opening and closing (kai he) are used in combination in a simple manipulation.

## Method

Take hold of the needle and give it a short lifting and thrusting movement of around 1–2 mm, following the principle of the ancient texts: 'Lift forcefully, thrust gently'.

In this technique, the pincer formed by the thumb and index finger is used only to steady and control the needle. *The active movement 'lifting forcefully'* relies on the action of the hand and not on that of the pincer formed by the fingers.

With the wrist locked in position, the right hand rests completely on the pad of the third finger, springing up smoothly through the intermediary of the proximal interphalangeal joint (PIP), which acts as a spring.

Join the upward and downward movements of the needle together into one continuous, even and harmonious sequence for the duration of the treatment, usually 10–15 seconds.

Withdraw the needle in one movement, either by raising it slowly and smoothly until it is out, or by lifting it slowly and smoothly in a spiral movement to widen the hole. Do not touch the point once the needle is out. The choice of withdrawal procedure is determined by the progress of the treatment.

## 3. REINFORCING BY ROTATION (Nian Zhuan)

In this technique the *Reinforcing* elements of slow and fast (xu ji), rotation (nian zhuan), nine and six (jiu liu), scratching (gua) and opening and closing (kai he) are used in combination in a simple manipulation.

### Method

Take hold of the needle (Figs 5.6, 5.7) and abruptly rotate it anti-clockwise through 45–90° (Fig. 5.8), pulling your thumb towards you then putting it back in position. The sequence starts with the thumb pulling backwards and finishes as it extends forwards. Repeat this movement to and fro 9 times or a multiple of 9 times.

Next, with the 'tiger claw' firmly in place, place the pad of your left third finger on top of the needle, holding it in place so it does not bend or penetrate deeper.

With the nail of your right index finger scratch downwards on the handle 9 times or a multiple of 9 times, taking care not to push the needle in deeper. The pressure of your left index finger against the base of the needle should prevent this (Fig. 5.9).

Withdraw the needle in two steps:

a. Quickly lift the needle up till the tip is just beneath the skin and hold it there for a fraction of a second.

b. Pull the needle out rapidly and massage the point with your left index finger.

## 4. REDUCING BY ROTATION (Nian Zhuan)

In this technique the *Reducing* elements of rotation (nian zhuan), nine and six (jiu liu), scratching (gua) and opening and closing (kai he) are used in combination in a simple manipulation.

### Method

Take hold of the needle and rotate it clockwise through 180–360° extending your thumb away from you then putting it back in position. The

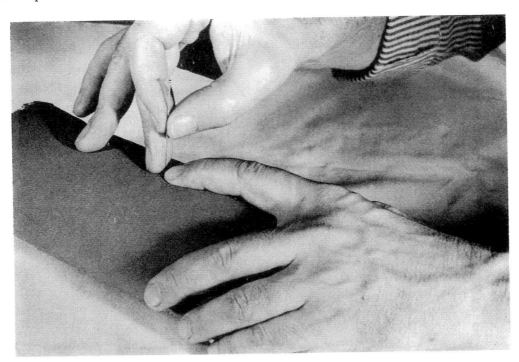

**Fig. 5.6**  Rotating to reinforce. Position of fingers before manipulation.

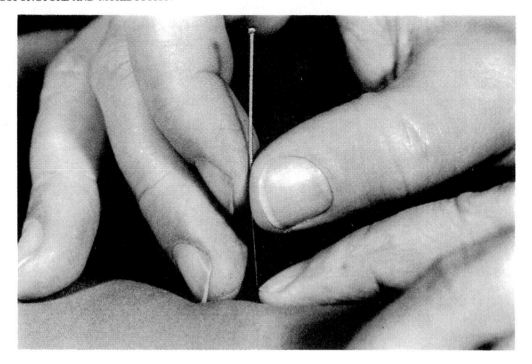

**Fig. 5.7** Enlarged view of same position.

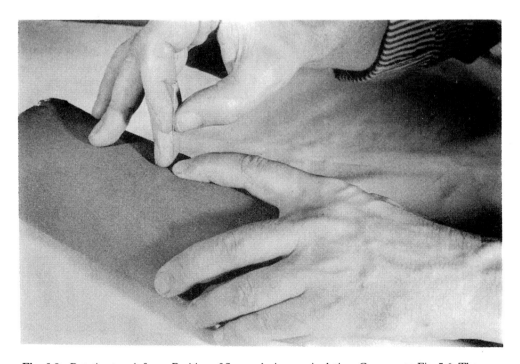

**Fig. 5.8** Rotating to reinforce. Position of fingers during manipulation. Compare to Fig. 5.6. The thumb has been pulled back.

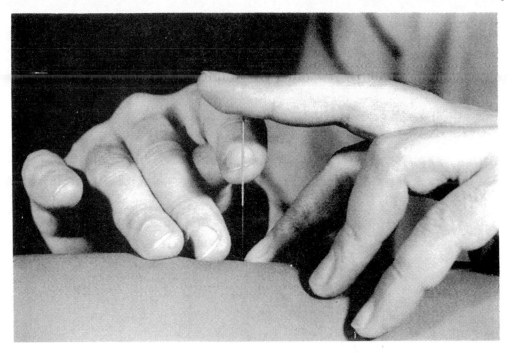

**Fig. 5.9**    Scratching downwards with the nail of the right index finger.

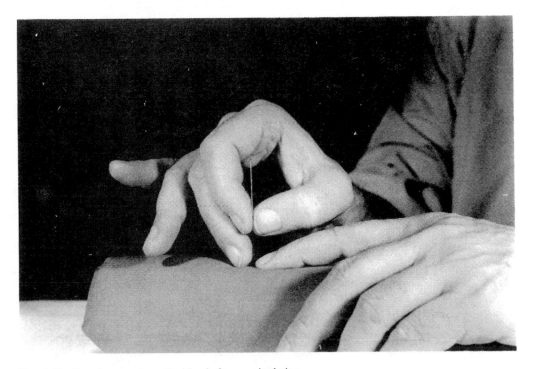

**Fig. 5.10**    Rotating to reduce. Position before manipulation.

sequence starts with the thumb extending forwards and finishes as it pulls back (Figs. 5.10–5.12).

Repeat this to-and-fro movement 6 times or a multiple of 6 times.

Next, with the 'tiger claw' firmly in place, place the pad of your left third finger on top of the needle, holding it in place so it does not bend or penetrate deeper.

With the nail of your right index finger scratch upwards on the handle 6 times or a multiple of 6 times, taking care not to pull the needle up. The pressure of the left index finger against the base of the needle should prevent this.

Withdraw the needle in one movement, either by raising it slowly and smoothly until it is out, or by lifting it slowly and smoothly in a spiral movement to widen the hole. Do not touch the point once the needle is out.

When the needle has been raised to just below the skin, make sure it is not caught up in any muscular fibres by giving it a small rotation to disengage it.

## 5. BALANCING (Ping Bu Ping Xie)

*Balancing*, Ping Bu Ping Xie (half reinforcing, half reducing or reinforcing and reducing equally) is, as its name indicates, a combination of reinforcing and reducing by rotation joined with reinforcing and reducing by lifting and thrusting.

This technique can also be used to obtain Qi.

### *Method*

Take hold of the needle and rotate it smoothly anti-clockwise 2 or 3 times, pulling your thumb towards you while thrusting the needle in about 5 mm. Next, rotate it the same number of times in the opposite direction whilst lifting it.

Continue these movements for a few seconds in *a continuous, even and harmonious sequence*. Withdraw the needle rapidly in one movement and do not touch the point afterwards.

## B. COMPLEX MANIPULATIONS

### 6. 'LIGHTING THE FIRE ON THE MOUNTAIN' (Shao Shan Huo)

This technique obtains a very strong reaction. The *Reinforcing* elements of slow and fast (xu ji), lifting and thrusting (ti cha) or rotation (nian zhuan),

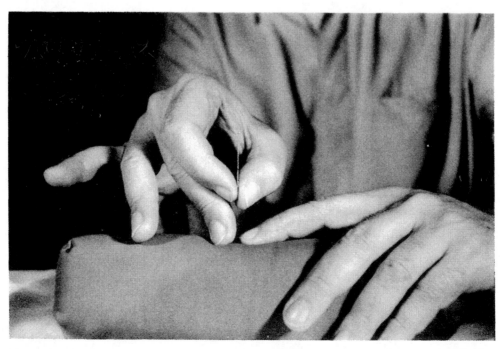

**Fig. 5.11** Rotating to reduce. Position during manipulation. Note extension of thumb and compare to Figs 5.8 and 5.10.

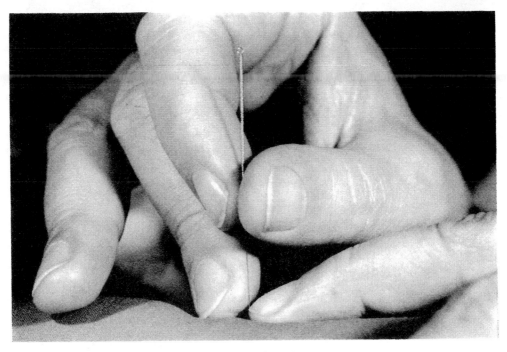

**Fig. 5.12** Enlarged view of Fig. 5.11 and extension of thumb.

advancing and withdrawing (jin tui), nine and six (jiu liu) and opening and closing (kai he) are used in combination in a complex manipulation.

Traditionally it is said to pull the Yang Qi down to meet the Yin Qi. It is commonly accompanied by a sensation of warmth or by sweating. It should only be used on thickly muscled areas, for example the limbs or the lumbar region.

This manipulation can also be used to obtain Qi.

### Method

Take hold of the needle and abruptly rotate it anti-clockwise through approximately 90°, pulling your thumb towards you then putting it back in position.

Repeat this movement to and fro 9 times or a multiple of 9 times; the needle is now at the 'preparatory' level.

With the 'tiger claw' held firmly, move your thumb and index finger no more than 2 mm up the handle, without breaking contact with the needle.

*NB: only the fingers should slide up, not the needle.*

Thrust the needle in slowly and forcefully no more than 2 mm and start the previous rotation procedure once again. The needle is now at the first level.

With the 'tiger claw' held firmly, move your thumb and index finger no more than 2 mm up the handle, without breaking contact with the needle. Thrust the needle in slowly and forcefully no more than 2 mm and start the previous rotation procedure once again. The needle is now at the second level.

With the 'tiger claw' held firmly, move your thumb and index finger no more than 2 mm up the handle, without breaking contact with the needle. Thrust the needle in slowly and forcefully no more than 2 mm and start the previous rotation procedure once again. The needle is now at the third level.

In the course of this manipulation the needle goes no deeper than 6 mm and undergoes 4 series of 9 rotations (nian zhuan).

With the 'tiger claw' held firmly, move your thumb and index finger down along the handle of the needle to the junction of the handle and the body. Take hold of the needle and lift it in one movement to the preparatory level.

Withdraw the needle in two steps:

a. Quickly lift the needle up till the tip is just beneath the skin and hold it there for a fraction of a second.

b. Pull the needle out rapidly and massage the point with your left index finger or thumb.

## Variations

A. Perform the entire manipulation as described, but replace rotation (nian zhuan) with lifting and thrusting to reinforce (ti cha) at each level, i.e. the needle is lifted and thrust 9 times at each level. This technique is the classical version of Shao Shan Huo (Fig. 5.13).

B. Perform the entire manipulation in exactly the same way as before, but replace reinforcing by rotation with 'green tortoise seeks the point', moving your hand up and down 9 times, like the boom of a pump on an oilwell (see technique 10 below).

## Associated diseases

Shao Shan Huo nourishes the Yuan Qi of the organs and is used to treat Empty and Cold diseases, such as stroke (Zhong Feng), leakages from defi-

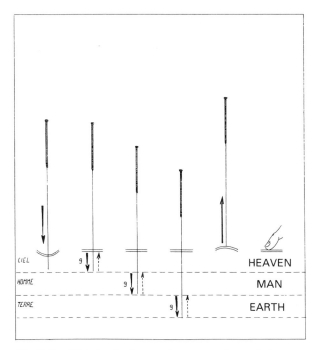

**Fig. 5.13** 'Lighting the fire on the mountain': classical version of Shao Shan Huo.

ciency of Qi, paraesthesia and paralysis, Wind and Damp Bi, cold limbs, diarrhoea, impotence, hernia, abdominal and lumbar pains.

This technique can be used to clear the Surface by inducing sweating in attacks of Wind or Cold. *Examples:*

● Using this technique on Zhongwan Ren 12 induces a sensation of warmth in the stomach and eliminates abdominal pains arising from Cold.

● Needle Fengchi GB 20 and Hegu LI 4 to induce sweating and clear the Surface.

● Needle Zusanli ST 36, Liangqiu ST 34 and Eye of the knee Xiyan (extra) to warm and disperse Cold and Damp and treat inflammation of the knee joint arising from Wind, Cold and Damp.

## 7. 'COOLNESS FROM HEAVEN' (Tou Tian Liang)

This technique, also known as 'Drawing down coolness from heaven', obtains a powerful reaction. The *Reducing* elements of slow and fast (xu ji), lifting and thrusting (ti cha) or rotation (nian zhuan), advancing and withdrawing (jin tui), nine and six (jiu liu) and opening and closing (kai he) are used in combination in a complex manipulation.

This technique should only be used on thickly muscled areas, for example the limbs or the lumbar region.

It is commonly accompanied by a sensation of cold.

## Method

Take hold of the needle and move your thumb and index finger about 6 mm up the handle without breaking contact.

*NB: only the fingers should slide up, not the needle.* In one movement thrust the needle in approximately 6 mm deeper. Rotate the needle clockwise through a large angle of 180–360°, extending your thumb away from you then pulling it back in position. Repeat this movement to and fro 6 times; the needle is now at the 'preparatory' level.

With the 'tiger claw' held firmly, move your thumb and index finger no more than 2 mm down the handle without breaking contact with the needle.

*NB: only the fingers should slide down, not the needle.*

Slowly and forcefully withdraw the needle about 2 mm. Rotate the needle clockwise through a large angle of 180–360°, extending your thumb away from you then pulling it back in position. Repeat this movement to and fro 6 times; the needle is now at the first level.

With the 'tiger claw' held firmly, move your thumb and index finger no more than 2 mm down the handle without breaking contact with the needle.

Slowly and forcefully withdraw the needle about 2 mm. Rotate the needle clockwise through a large angle of 180–360°, extending your thumb away from you then pulling it back in position. Repeat this movement to and fro 6 times; the needle is now at the second level.

With the 'tiger claw' held firmly, move your thumb and index finger no more than 2 mm down the handle without breaking contact with the needle.

Slowly and forcefully withdraw the needle about 2 mm. Rotate the needle clockwise through a large angle of 180–360°, extending your thumb away from you then pulling it back in position. Repeat this movement to and fro 6 times; the needle is now at the third level.

In the course of this manipulation the needle is

withdrawn 6 mm and undergoes 4 series of 6 rotations (nian zhuan).

Withdraw the needle in one movement, either by raising it slowly and smoothly until it is out, or by lifting it slowly and smoothly in a spiral movement to widen the hole. Do not touch the point once the needle is out.

### Variations

A. Perform the entire manipulation as described, but replace rotation with lifting and thrusting to reduce (ti cha), raising and lowering the needle 6 times at each level. This variation of Tou Tian Liang is considered the classical technique (Fig. 5.14).

B. Perform the entire manipulation as described, but follow the 6 rotations (nian zhuan) with 6 lifting and thrusting movements (ti cha).

### Associated diseases

Tou Tian Liang disperses excess Yang, expels perverse energy and treats diseases arising from Fullness and Heat such as spastic stroke (closed Zhong Feng), sunstroke, hyperpyrexia, verbal delirium, madness, epistaxis, swelling of the gums, body heat, dry stools.

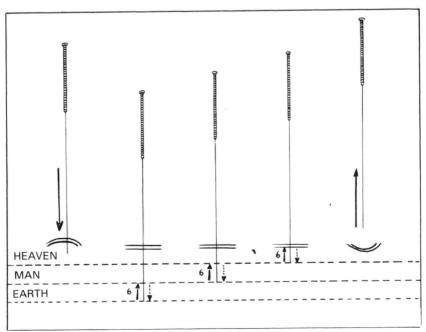

**Fig. 5.14** 'Coolness from heaven': classical version of Tou Tian Liang.

This technique is also used in attacks of external Wind Heat to cool Heat and clear the Surface.

*Examples:*

• Needle Zhongfeng LIV 4 to treat conjunctivitis.

• Needle Shuidao ST 28, Zhongji Ren 3 and Filiu KI 7 to disperse Heat, increase urination and treat retention of urine arising from Fullness of Heat in the Bladder.

• Needle Dazhui Du 14, Feishui BL 13, Hegu LI 4 to cool Heat and clear the Surface to treat fever arising from external Wind Heat.

## 8. REINFORCING BY OBTAINING SENSATIONS OF HEAT

This technique is also known as 'Reinforcing by making Heat penetrate' (Jing Re Bu Fa). The *Reinforcing* elements of slow and fast (xu ji), rotation (nian zhuan) or lifting and thrusting (ti cha), advancing and withdrawing (jin tui), nine and six (jiu liu), rotation (cuo nian), scratching (gua), breathing (hu xi), and opening and closing (kai he) are used in combination in a complex manipulation.

### Method

Take hold of the needle and abruptly rotate it anti-clockwise through approximately 90°, pulling your thumb towards you then putting it back in position. Repeat this movement to and fro 9 times or a multiple of 9 times; the needle is now at the 'preparatory' level.

With the 'tiger claw' held firmly, move your thumb and index finger no more than 2 mm up the handle, without breaking contact with the needle.

*NB: only the fingers should slide up, not the needle.*

Thrust the needle in slowly and forcefully no more than 2 mm and start the previous rotation procedure once again. The needle is now at the first level.

With the 'tiger 'claw' held firmly, move your thumb and index finger no more than 2 mm up the handle, without breaking contact with the needle. Thrust the needle in slowly and forcefully no more than 2 mm and start the previous rotation proce-

dure once again. The needle is now at the second level.

With the 'tiger claw' held firmly, move your thumb and index finger no more than 2 mm up the handle, without breaking contact with the needle. Thrust the needle in slowly and forcefully no more than 2 mm and start the previous rotation procedure once again. The needle is now at the third level.

In the course of this manipulation the needle goes no deeper than 6 mm and undergoes 4 series of 9 rotations (nian zhuan).

Push the needle a fraction of a millimetre deeper and rotate it to reinforce, entwining the fibres of tissue until the needle is gripped firmly (cuo nian). Next place the third finger of your left hand on top of the needle and scratch it downwards 9 times with the nail of your right index finger (gua).

Withdrawing the needle: unwind the fibres of tissue and withdraw the needle in two steps:

a. Quickly lift the needle up till the tip is just beneath the skin and hold it there for a fraction of a second.

b. Pull the needle out rapidly and massage the point with your left index finger or thumb.

### Clinical practice

— This manipulation can be augmented by adding the reinforcing element of breathing (hu xi). Ask the patient to breathe out through the mouth during the 4 series of 9 reinforcing rotations.

— The patient should feel a sensation of heat during or after the scratching. As soon as this sensation is felt the procedure should be stopped and should not be repeated. If no heat is sensed in the 20–40 seconds following the scratching, the technique should be abandoned.

— Do not confuse the sensation of heat arising from correct technique with the same sensation obtained by mistake when a small vessel (arteriole) is damaged by the insertion or manipulation of the needle.

### Variations

1. Replace reinforcing by rotation (nian zhuan) with lifting and thrusting (ti cha). In this case

breathing is integrated as follows: the patient breathes in through the nose and breathes out through the mouth. The needle is pushed in whilst the patient breathes out and withdrawn whilst he breathes in.

2. Take hold of the needle and obtain Qi, then apply the 'tiger claw' more forcefully, rotating the needle to reinforce 9 times (nian zhuan), followed by lifting and thrusting to reinforce 9 times (ti cha). Finish with another 9 rotations to reinforce (nian zhuan), and withdraw the needle using the method described above.

### Associated diseases

Flaccid stroke (open Zhong Feng) with symptoms of exhaustion, paraesthesia and chronic paralysis, polyuria, loose stools, borborygmus, diarrhoea, lumbar pains, impotence, nocturnal emission, and Wind or Damp Bi arising from Emptiness and Cold.

This technique is also used in chronic diseases and on patients with a weak constitution.

*Examples:*

● Needle Shenshu BL 23, Zhibian BL 49, Fengshi GB 31, Yinshi ST 33, Xuehai SP 10, Zusanli ST 36, Sanyinjiao SP 6 for the sequelae of poliomyelitis in children, to benefit the circulation in the channels and collaterals by warming.

● Needle Zhongwan Ren 12, Tianshu ST 25, Qihai Ren 6, Yaoshu Du 2, Huiyang BL 35 to treat abdominal pain and loose stools arising from Emptiness and Cold by warming.

## 9. REDUCING BY OBTAINING SENSATIONS OF COLD

This technique is also known as 'Reducing by making Water penetrate' (Jin Shui Xie Fa). The *Reducing* elements of slow and fast (xu ji), rotation (nian zhuan) or lifting and thrusting (ti cha), advancing and withdrawing (jin tui), nine and six (jiu liu), rotation (cuo nian), scratching (gua), breathing (hu xi) and opening and closing (kai he) are used in combination in a complex manipulation.

### Method

Take hold of the needle and move your thumb and index finger about 6 mm up the handle without breaking contact.

*NB: only the fingers should slide up, not the needle.* In one movement thrust the needle in approximately 6 mm deeper. Rotate the needle clockwise through a large angle of 180–360°, extending your thumb away from you then pulling it back in position. Repeat this movement to and fro 6 times; the needle is now at the 'preparatory' level.

With the 'tiger claw' held firmly, move your thumb and index finger no more than 2 mm down the handle without breaking contact with the needle.

*NB: only the fingers should slide down, not the needle.*

Slowly and forcefully withdraw the needle about 2 mm. Rotate the needle clockwise through a large angle of 180–360°, extending your thumb away from you then pulling it back in position. Repeat this movement to and fro 6 times; the needle is now at the first level.

With the 'tiger claw' held firmly, move your thumb and index finger no more than 2 mm down the handle without breaking contact with the needle.

Slowly and forcefully withdraw the needle about 2 mm. Rotate the needle clockwise through a large angle of 180–360°, extending your thumb away from you then pulling it back in position. Repeat this movement to and fro 6 times; the needle is now at the second level.

With the 'tiger claw' held firmly, move your thumb and index finger no more than 2 mm down the handle without breaking contact with the needle.

Slowly and forcefully withdraw the needle about 2 mm. Rotate the needle clockwise through a large angle of 180–360°, extending your thumb away from you then pulling it back in position. Repeat this movement to and fro 6 times; the needle is now at the third level.

In the course of this manipulation the needle is withdrawn no more than 6 mm and undergoes 4 series of 6 rotations.

With the 'tiger claw' held firmly, and in one movement, thrust the needle in once more to a depth of approximately 6 mm, as if starting the entire reducing technique all over again. Once at the 'preparatory' level, however, withdraw the needle a fraction of a millimetre and rotate it to reduce, entwining the fibres of tissue until the needle is gripped firmly (cuo nian). Next, place the third finger of your left hand on top of the needle and scratch it upwards 6 times with the nail of your right index finger (gua).

Withdraw the needle in one movement, either by raising it slowly and smoothly until it is out, or by lifting it slowly and smoothly in a spiral movement to widen the hole. Do not touch the point once the needle is out.

### Clinical practice

— The manipulation can be augmented by adding the reducing element of breathing (hu xi). Ask the patient to breathe in through the nose during the 4 series of 6 reducing rotations.

— Before withdrawing the needle, it is important to make sure it is not caught up in any muscular fibres by giving it a small rotation in the opposite direction to disengage it.

— The patient should feel a sensation of coolness or icy cold during or after the scratching. As soon as this sensation is felt the procedure should be stopped. If no sensation of cold is sensed in the 20–40 seconds following the scratching, the technique should be abandoned.

— Do not confuse the sensation of cold arising from correct technique with the same sensation obtained by mistake when a small vessel (vein) is damaged by the insertion or manipulation of the needle.

### Variations

1. Replace reducing by rotation (nian zhuan) with lifting and thrusting. Breathing is incorporated as follows: the patient breathes in through the nose and breathes out through the mouth. The needle is pushed in whilst the patient breathes in, and withdrawn whilst he breathes out.

2. Take hold of the needle and obtain Qi, then relax 'tiger claw' a little, rotating the needle to reduce 6 times (nian zhuan), followed by lifting and thrusting (ti cha) to reduce 6 times. Finish with another 6 rotations to reduce (nian zhuan), and withdraw the needle using the method described above.

### Associated diseases

Spastic stroke (closed Zhong Feng), hyperpyrexia,

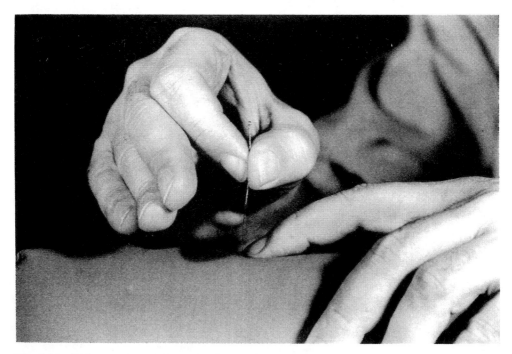

**Fig. 5.15** 'Flying away' to reinforce. Starting position.

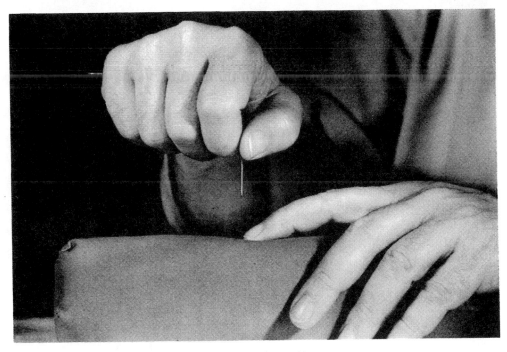

**Fig. 5.16** 'Flying away' to reinforce. Alternative starting position.

sunstroke, red eyes, ulceration of the lips, oppression of the chest, dry stools, constipation, verbal delirium, and madness, arising from Full Heat.

*Examples:*

● Needle Dachangshu BL 25, Tianshu ST 25, Zusanli ST 36, Fenglong ST 40 to treat dry constipation by cooling Heat and purging the bowels.

● Needle Jiache ST 6, Yifeng TB 17, Hegu LI 4 to disperse swellings caused by mumps, by cooling Heat and creating Cold.

## 10. 'GREEN TORTOISE SEEKS THE POINT' (Cang Gui Tan Xue)

According to the classics, this Reinforcing technique should be used on each of the main points of the treatment in succession. In practice, the sequence of needling follows one direction, depending on where the acupuncturist is standing in relation to the patient.

This manipulation can also be used to obtain Qi.

### Method

Take hold of the needle and use lifting and thrusting at a depth of approximately 2 mm. At the same time move the needle forwards and backwards in a circular movement in the vertical plane. This manipulation is carried out by moving the pincer formed by the index finger and thumb like the boom of an oilwell pump.

Continue the manipulation until Qi is obtained (no more than a minute). If the aim is to stimulate the point, carry on for as long as the treatment requires.

## 11. FLYING AWAY (Fei)

Flying away is a powerful Reinforcing and Reducing technique used for intense pain. It is applied differently depending on whether the patient has a tendency towards obesity or skinniness and emaciation.

### Method

*Reinforcing.* Take hold of the needle and grip it tightly between the tips of your index finger and thumb (Figs 5.15, 5.16). Next snap your index finger away suddenly, as if you were flicking it at something. At the same time move your third finger away from the cushion and open your hand out wide, fingers apart.

a

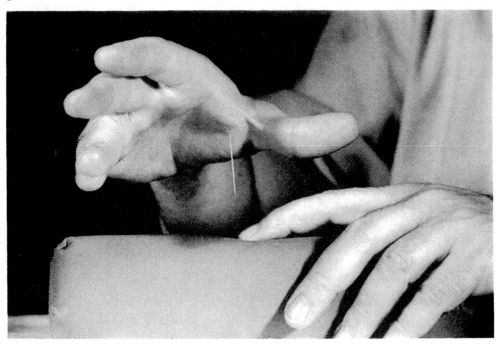

b

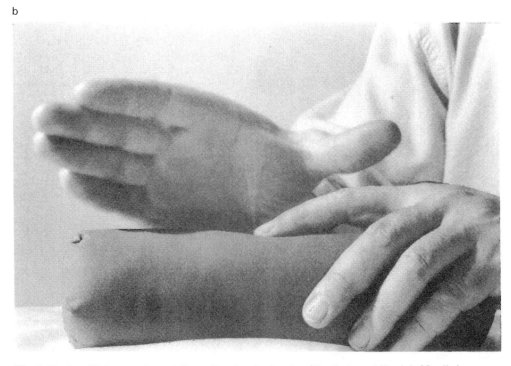

**Fig. 5.17a, b** 'Flying away' to reinforce. Opening the hand. **a** Needle immobilised. **b** Needle in motion.

The needle is left vibrating strongly on its own, oscillating visibly. The more pronounced the oscillation, the stronger the effect (Fig. 5.17a, b).

*Reducing.* Take hold of the needle and grip it tightly between the tips of your thumb and index finger. Next snap your thumb away suddenly, as if you were flicking it at something. At the same time move your third finger away from the cushion and open your hand out wide, fingers apart. This time, however, the proximal and distal interphalangeal joints of the index finger remain partially flexed (Fig. 5.18).

The needle is left vibrating strongly on its own, oscillating visibly. The more pronounced the oscillation, the stronger the effect.

### Clinical practice

— With obese patients with Emptiness of energy, start off by giving the needle one anti-clockwise reinforcing rotation (Bu), then one clockwise reducing rotation (Xie). Pause for a fraction of a second and then continue with reinforcing Fei technique. The two techniques combined should be performed in one sequence.

— With thin or emaciated patients start off by giving the needle one clockwise reducing rotation (Xie), followed by one anti-clockwise reinforcing rotation (Bu). Pause for a fraction of a second, gripping the needle tightly, then proceed with reducing Fei technique. The two techniques combined should be performed in one sequence.

## 12. 'GREEN DRAGON SWINGS HIS TAIL' (Cang Long Yao Wei)

This technique is a powerful way of moving Qi to the site of the disease and is used to treat severe pain. The *Zhen Jiu Da Cheng* states that this manipulation 'Reinforces Emptiness and Diffuses Warmth' (Bu Fa He Wen San Fa).

'Green dragon swings his tail' uses swinging and shaking (yao), nine and six (jiu liu), opening and closing (kai he), and sometimes blocking (guan bi) and breathing (hu xi) in combination.

### Method

Place the cushion in front of you, *its centre directly in front of the left axillary line of the body.*

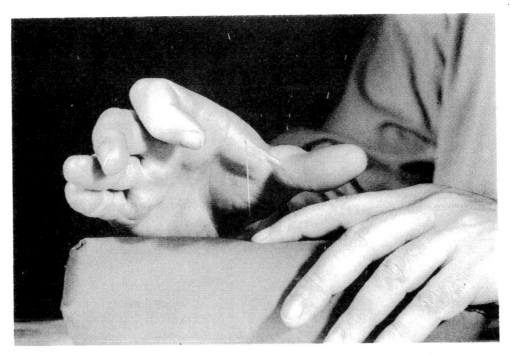

**Fig. 5.18** 'Flying away' to reduce. If the manipulation is performed correctly the only difference is that the index finger is kept flexed.

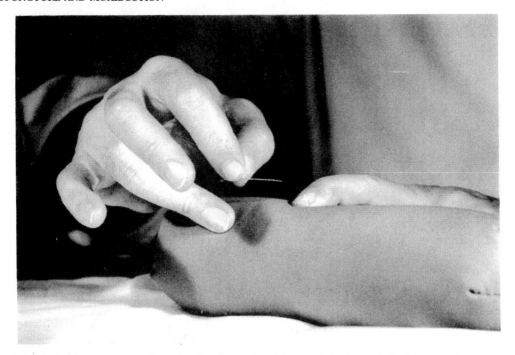

**Fig. 5.19** 'Green dragon swings his tail'. The handle of the needle lies beneath the left index finger. The angle formed by the pads of the right index finger and thumb retains the end of the handle in place.

Insert the needle perpendicularly to an appropriate depth, i.e. 1.2 cm.

Assuming that the site of the pain is on the left-hand edge of the cushion, place your left index finger to the right of the needle and press firmly (if the practitioner is facing south the finger is placed west of the needle).

*Put your right thumb and index finger together in a pincer and wedge the end of the handle of the needle into the distal angle formed by the fingertips. The needle should not be gripped firmly, merely held in place* (Fig. 5.19).

Bend the handle of the needle over, your index fingernail underneath, until it is parallel to the surface of the cushion, pointing along its central axis.

Place the fourth finger of your right hand on the side of the cushion. The tip of the needle is now pointing towards the site of the disease.

Using your fourth finger to lean on, shake the handle up and down vertically to the axis of the cushion. Do this 9 or a multiple of 9 times, as if 'plying a scull'. The left index finger remains beneath the needle, on the same side as the handle, never on the opposite side, so that the

Qi can move towards the site of the disease (Fig. 5.20).

Withdraw the needle swiftly and massage the point.

### Clinical practice

— Use this technique on a point far enough away from the affected area so that you can launch the Qi at it from a distance.

— Continue the manipulation until the Qi moves, but never exceed one minute.

— If the Qi consistently refuses to move, it can be mobilised by massaging the pathway of the channel with the left hand, starting from the point and working towards the area to be treated.

### Variation

The left index finger is placed behind the needle (north) instead of to the right (west). The manipulation is performed in exactly the same way as above, keeping the needle curved along the axis of the cushion, thus enabling Qi to move in both directions if desired.

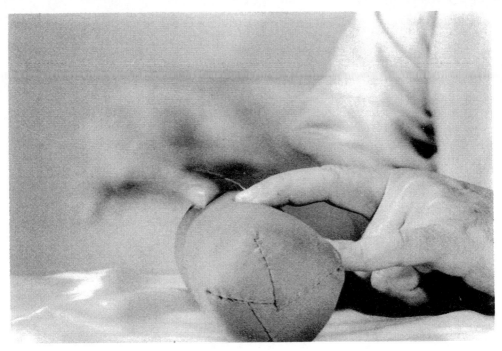

**Fig. 5.20** 'Green dragon swings his tail.' The right hand rests on the fourth finger and moves the needle perpendicularly to the axis of the cushion, as if 'plying a scull'.

### Associated diseases

False or real masses and accumulations in the Middle or Lower Heaters (Zheng Jia Ji Ju), tuberculous lymph nodes, goitre, painful articular swelling, all arising from stasis of Qi and Blood.
*Example:*

● In cases of abdominal pain arising from stasis of Qi and Blood, use this technique to needle Zhongwan Ren 12, Tianshu ST 25, Guanyuan Ren 4, Zusanli ST 36 and Sanyinjiao SP 6, to warm and move Qi and Blood and help disperse stagnation.

### 13. 'WHITE TIGER SHAKES HIS HEAD' (Bai Hu Yao Tou)

This technique is also called 'red phoenix shakes his head', and is a powerful way of circulating Qi. It is used to launch Qi from a distance towards the site of the disease, striking it like the bolt of a crossbow. The *Zhen Jiu Da Cheng* classifies it as a Reducing technique (Xie Fa).

'White tiger shakes his head' uses lifting and thrusting (ti cha), swinging and shaking (yao), nine and six (jiu liu), blocking (guan bi), breathing (hu xi) and rotation (nian zhuan) in combination.

### Method

Place the cushion in front of you, *its centre directly in front of the left axillary line of the body.*

Insert the needle perpendicularly to an appropriate depth, i.e. 1.2 cm.

Assuming that the site of the pain is on the left-hand edge of the cushion, place your left index finger behind the needle, i.e. to the north of the needle, if the practitioner faces south. Place your right hand to the west of the needle, at 45° to the axis of the cushion, balancing on the hypothenar eminence.

Hold the needle with your right hand, using three fingers (thumb, index and third finger), and bend the needle over at right angles to the axis of the cushion.

As the needle is inclined over the left index finger, extend your right thumb outwards while thrusting the needle in slightly deeper (Fig. 5.21).

Swing the needle in the other direction, pulling your thumb back and withdrawing the needle

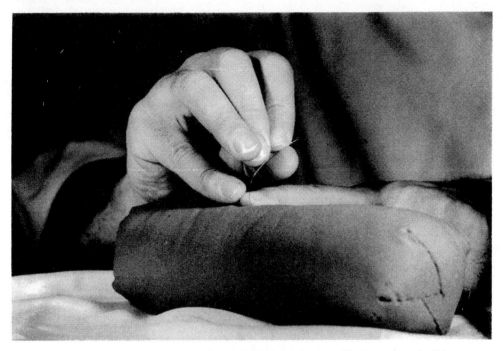

**Fig. 5.21**   'White tiger shakes his head.' The left index finger is perpendicular to the axis of the cushion. Note the position of the thumb, index and third fingers of the right hand holding the needle. The thumb is extended as they lean over towards the left index finger.

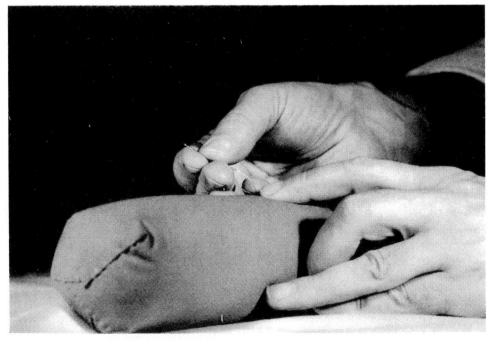

**Fig. 5.22**   'White tiger shakes his head.' Note the right thumb has been pulled back, and the left index finger is perpendicular to the axis of the cushion.

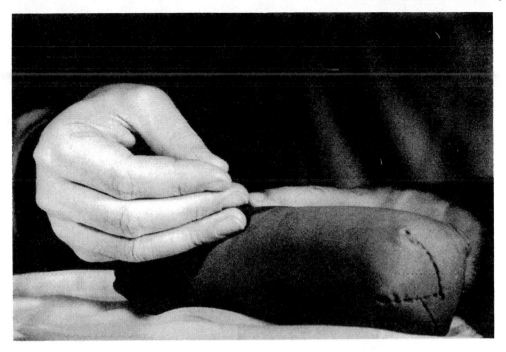

**Fig. 5.23**   'White tiger shakes his head.' Same position as in Fig. 5.22, seen from another angle.

slightly (Figs 5.22, 5.23). Continue swinging the needle gently from side to side 6 times or a multiple of 6 times.

Withdraw the needle slowly and do not touch the point afterwards.

### Clinical practice

— This technique can be used in combination with breathing (hu xi). Ask the patient to breathe naturally, exhaling through the nose and inhaling through the mouth. The reducing movement (extending the thumb) should stop whilst the patient is breathing out.

— Use this technique on a point sufficiently far away from the affected area.

— The manipulation should continue until Qi is felt along the channel, but should never exceed one minute.

— If the Qi consistently refuses to move, it can be mobilised by massaging the pathway of the channel with the left hand, starting from the point and working towards the area to be treated.

### Associated diseases

Loss of consciousness, verbal delirium, agitation

and anxiety with sensation of heat in the chest, madness, stagnation and constriction in the channels and collaterals, spasms, and stiff neck arising from Fullness and Heat.

*Examples:*

● Needle Hegu LI 4, Renzhong Du 26, Fenglong ST 40 with this technique to treat 'agitated madness' type diseases by expelling Wind, transforming phlegm, and expanding the 'openings'[1].

## 14. YIN HIDDEN IN YANG (Yang Zhong Yin Yin Fa)

This technique combines Reinforcing with Reducing. 'Reinforcing is Yang, Reducing is Yin.' The term 'Yin hidden in Yang' implies that whilst the technique is reinforcing it also contains an element which is reducing.

Reinforcing on the Exterior is followed by reducing in the Interior. This is accomplished by combining slow and fast (xu ji), lifting and thrusting (ti cha) and nine and six (jiu liu). Exterior refers to the needle when it is inserted to half

---

[1] 'Openings': the Liver opens into the eyes, the Kidneys open into the ears etc.

the required depth of the point; Interior refers to the needle when it is inserted to the full depth of the point.

## Method

If the required depth of insertion is 1 cun, start by inserting the needle to a depth of 5 fen, then use lifting and thrusting 9 times or a multiple of 9 times, thrusting slowly and forcefully, lifting swiftly and gently.

Next insert the needle to 1 cun, then use lifting and thrusting 6 times or a multiple of 6 times, thrusting swiftly and gently, lifting slowly and forcefully.

Withdraw the needle (Fig. 5.24).

## Clinical practice

The patient should be able to detect a sensation of warmth around the needle after the sequence of reinforcing movements, then a sensation of coolness after the sequence of reducing movements.

## Associated diseases

This method consists of reinforcing followed by reducing and is therefore suitable for the treatment of Cold diseases which contain an element of Heat, or Empty diseases which contain an element of Fullness.

*Example:*

• A patient has degenerative paraplegia, has been bedridden for a long time, and suffers from urinary tract infection. He has daily episodes of hyperpyrexia and shivering. This is an example of Fullness within Emptiness or Heat within Cold. This condition could be treated by needling Quchi LI 11, Hegu LI 4, Zhongji Ren 3 and Sanyinjiao SP 6 with this technique.

## 15. YANG HIDDEN IN YIN (Yin Zhong Yin Yang Fa)

This technique combines Reinforcing with Reducing in the same way as the one above. 'Reinforcing is Yang, Reducing is Yin.' The term 'Yang hidden in Yin' implies that whilst the technique is

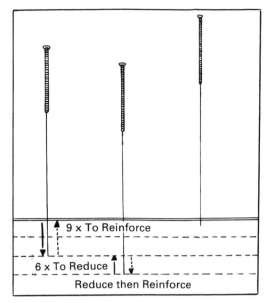

**Fig. 5.24** 'Yin hidden in Yang': reinforce first, then reduce.

reducing, it also contains an element which is reinforcing.

Reducing in the interior is followed by reinforcing on the surface, using slow and fast (xu ji), lifting and thrusting (ti cha) and nine and six (jiu liu) in combination.

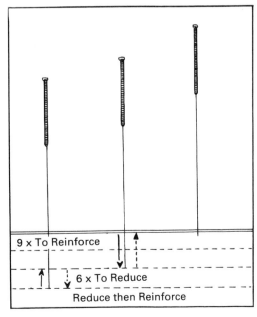

**Fig. 5.25** 'Yang hidden in Yin': reduce first, then reinforce.

## Method

If the required depth of insertion is 1 cun, insert the needle and gently bring it to this depth. Keep the needle at this depth and start reducing by thrusting swiftly and gently, lifting slowly and forcefully. Perform this manipulation 6 times or a multiple of 6 times.

Next withdraw the needle to a depth of 5 fen and start reinforcing by thrusting slowly and forcefully, and lifting swiftly and gently. The movement is repeated 9 times or a multiple of 9 times.

Withdraw the needle (Fig. 5.25).

## Clinical practice

The patient should be able to detect a sensation of coolness around the needle after the sequence of reducing movements, then a sensation of warmth after the sequence of reinforcing movements.

## Associated diseases

This method consists of reducing followed by reinforcing and is therefore suitable for the treatment of Hot diseases which contain an element of Cold, or Full diseases which contain an element of Emptiness.

*Example:*

• A patient suffers from rheumatoid arthritis with perspiration and hyperpyrexia. When the fever drops, his joints are still painful, he is sensitive to Cold and Wind and needs to wrap himself up warmly. These are symptoms of 'Emptiness within Fullness' or signs of 'Cold within Heat'. The points should therefore be stimulated with this technique.

## 16.  'DRAGON AND TIGER COME TO BLOWS' (Long Hu Jiao Zhuan)

This mixed Reinforcing and Reducing technique is intended to stop pain and arises from the marriage of two simple techniques: rotation (nian zhuan) and nine and six (jiu liu). It is interesting to note that 'Dragon and tiger come to blows' is similar to 'Yang hidden in Yin' and 'Yin hidden in Yang' in the way the techniques are combined. According to Yang Ji Zhou, the latter are designed to treat both Cold and Heat, and balance Yin and Yang, which is why they use lifting and thrusting (ti cha). 'Dragon and tiger come to blows', on the other hand, is intended to stop pain by liberating Qi in the channels, and uses rotation (nian zhuan).

## Method

When needling points on the 3 arm Yang channels, the 3 leg Yin channels and on Ren Mai, the needle should be rotated 9 times to reinforce, which is called 'Dragon', followed by 6 more times to reduce, which is called 'Tiger'. When needling points on the 3 arm Yin channels, the 3 leg Yang and on Du Mai, the needle should be rotated 6 times to reduce, then 9 times to reinforce. This technique consists of alternating reinforcing (Dragon) with reducing (Tiger), hence the title 'Dragon and tiger come to blows'.

When practising on the cushion, simply alternate sequences of 9 rotations to reinforce with sequences of 6 rotations to reduce.

## Associated diseases

This technique is intended to circulate and regulate Qi in the channels, to circulate the Ying and the Wei. For this reason it is very effective in the treatment of pain.

# Moxibustion and other techniques

# 6. Moxibustion (Jiu Fa)

*Ling Shu*, Chapter 73:

If a condition does not respond to needling it should be treated with moxa.

*Yi Xue Ru Men:*

Moxa should be used on those conditions which do not respond to medication or acupuncture.

In the opinion of the authors, the term 'moxa' is derived from the Portuguese word *mechia*, or the Japanese word *mogusa* (a variety of mugwort). The term first came into use in the West in 1677.

Moxibustion is without doubt the most ancient form of therapy in China. The discovery of the *Treatise on moxibustion of the eleven vessels of Yin and Yang (Ying Yang Shi Yi Mai Jiu Jing)* in the tomb of Ma Wang (Ma Wang Dui), proves how much had already been learned about the use of moxa a thousand years before the Nei Jing.

References to the indications for moxibustion can be found in the ancient texts which followed the Treatise:

*Su Wen* (Ch. 12): '. . . cold in the organs gives rise to diseases of "repletion". These should be treated with moxa, which was discovered in the North'. (Ch. 74): 'If the condition is cold use heat'.

*Ling Shu* (Ch. 10): 'When Yang energy is weak in the Interior, manifesting in a weak pulse, the physician should use moxa'. (Ch. 48): 'Cold causes a blockage in the flow of blood and can be eliminated by heating with moxa'. 'For prolapse or loss of energy use moxa.'

*Shang Han Lun:* 'Use seven moxas on Shao Yang'.

*Zhen Jiu Da Cheng* (scroll 9): 'To maintain health San Li should never become dry' (see below: scarring moxibustion and indications for moxibustion).

These works also clarify the relation between moxibustion, acupuncture and herbalism:

*Ling Shu* (Ch. 73): 'When a disease cannot be treated by needling it should be treated with moxa'.

Yi Xue Ru Men: 'Moxa should be given to those who have not improved with medication or needling'.

The Chinese word for moxa is Jiu, which means 'burning'. Moxibustion is used to stimulate the acupuncture points by the combustion of different materials in order to regulate the physiological activity of the body.

The herb most often used is mugwort, but after the Jin and Tang eras the scope of moxibustion was broadened with the introduction of medicinal substances and mugwort in combination. Today, using the same basic principle, sunshine and electricity can both be used as a source of heat: all of these constitute moxa with heat (Huo Re Jiu).

Certain products or preparations, depending on their action, may be applied directly onto the acupuncture point. The vesicatory effect of the medication in direct contact with the skin produces a stimulation without heat. Similarly, cold itself is used as a means of stimulation: all of these come under the classification of moxa without heat.

Moxa with heat is the form of moxibustion most often used, usually with mugwort.

## MOXA WITH HEAT

### A. MOXA WITH MUGWORT

Mugwort (Aiye), *Artemisia vulgaris*, or *Artemisia*

*argyi*, is part of the Compositae family. It is a herbaceous perennial with a strong fragrance, and very common in France. In China the best varieties are found in Hubei, where the custom is to gather them during the Duan Yang festival, on the fifth day of the fifth lunar month (Fig. 6.1).[1]

Zhu Dan-xi (1280–1358), summarises the action of mugwort in one sentence: 'Its nature is extremely hot, making energy move downwards when taken internally, and upwards when used in moxa'.

## Internal use

### Properties:

- Acrid and bitter flavour,
- Hot nature,
- Enters the channels of the Lung, Liver, Spleen and Kidneys.

### Action:

- Warms the channels and stops bleeding,
- Disperses Cold and relieves pain,
- Stops cough, calms asthma and disperses Phlegm.

### Applications:

- Cold and Emptiness in the uterus,
- Abdominal pain during menstruation,
- Leucorrhoea,
- Lumbar pain,
- Oppression in the thorax and abdomen,
- Cough and asthma.

## External use

Ben Cao-jing says: 'Mugwort has a bitter flavour, its Qi is light and hot, and it is Yang within Yin. When used in moxa it can treat any disease'.

*Applications:* Action of mugwort in moxibustion:

---

[1] If the mugwort is gathered after this time (mid-May) its fragrance dissipates and it becomes less effective medicinally. The Chinese say 'If you wear mugwort in your hair you'll grow strong and nimble'. The properties of fresh mugwort are also known to Western writers: 'Artemisia et elelisphacum alligatas qui habeat viator, negatur lassitudinem sentire' (Pliny). 'If a footman takes mugwort and puts it into his shoes in the morning, he may go forty miles before noon, and not be weary' (Cole: *Art of Simpling*).

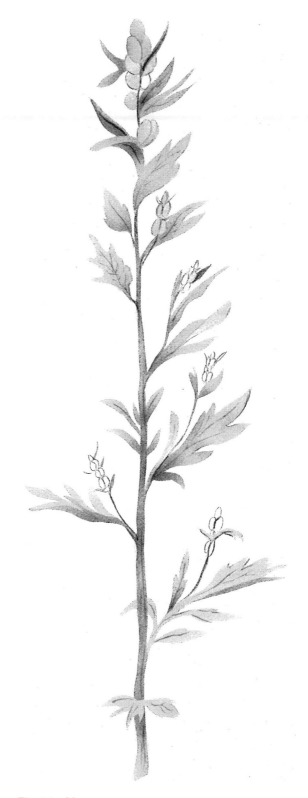

**Fig. 6.1**  Mugwort stem.

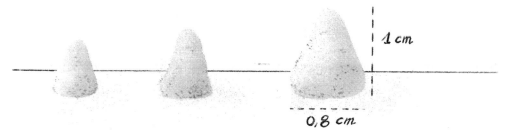

**Fig. 6.2**  Different sized cones of mugwort.

- warms and moves Qi and the Blood,
- strengthens Kidney Yang (Yuan Yang),
- expels Wind and disperses Cold,
- cools Heat and dispels toxins,
- invigorates the Blood and dissolves stagnation.

***Manufacture of moxa punk from mugwort.***
After harvesting, the leaves are removed from the stalks and branches, then dried. After drying they are crushed to a fine down, similar to cotton fibre, then passed through a comb to eliminate any impurities. For use in moxa cones, the punk needs to be even finer, so the leaf veins are removed by rolling the leaves in the palm of the hand. Care is taken not to damage the vegetable fibres so the cones remain firm.

Fresh moxa punk is greenish in colour, and highly inflammable. When used in moxibustion it causes intense pain. Old moxa punk has lost its oils and is yellow in colour. It maintains an even temperature during moxibustion (600° Celsius) and does not cause discomfort. It is therefore better to use the latter, as Meng Zi explains in the *Li Lou Pian*: 'A disease which has lasted for seven years should be treated with three year old mugwort'.

The best moxa punk is seven years old and yellow in colour. The sensation of heat caused by its moxibustion disappears and is replaced by a sensation of coolness similar to camphor. With fresh mugwort the sensation of heat persists.

The mugwort is kept in cloth sacks which are hung up. They must be dried out frequently to prevent mould, damp and damage from insects.

Moxibustion can be administered with the use of moxa cones or moxa sticks.

## MOXIBUSTION USING MOXA CONES

### Making moxa cones

Place a wad of moxa on a flat surface and shape it between your thumb, index and third fingers into small cones of different sizes.

The largest cones should be 1 cm high, 0.8 cm in diameter at the base and weigh roughly 1 g. The medium-sized cones are about the size of an olive stone, and the smallest are the size of a grain of corn. The latter are used for direct moxa (Fig. 6.2).

Cones can either be made from pure mugwort, or a blend of mugwort and medicinal substances. For example, take 90 g of old moxa punk, spray it with alcohol to moisten it and add 3 g of realgar (native arsenic sulphide) (see important note, p. 92). Mix well and knead together, then add 0.3 g of musk. Blend this in and shape into cones.

### General indications for cones

The size and quantity of cones used depends on the nature of the disease and the location of the area to be treated.

Large cones are used in larger quantities on places where there is plenty of muscle, e.g. the waist, back, abdomen, shoulders and thighs. Smaller cones are used where there is not so much muscle and the skin is thin, e.g. the back of the neck and the hands and feet.

The smallest number used is between 1 and 3. The classics say that the largest number is 'several hundred'.

In Empty and Cold conditions a large number of cones should be used.

Moxa should not be used in the initial stage of febrile diseases.

There are two moxibustion techniques using cones: the cone is put straight on to the skin (direct moxa), or it rests on something which is placed between it and the skin (indirect moxa). In both techniques the cone is lit from the top.

## Direct moxibustion

To make the cone stick to the surface of the skin, use a little alcohol for the medium-sized cones, and a little garlic juice for the small cones. Cut off the end of a clove of garlic and rub the skin with the open end. Bear in mind that garlic is an irritant and can sometimes cause blistering.

Direct moxibustion is an invasive procedure and can damage the skin. There are three kinds of moxibustion, classified by degree of invasiveness:

— non-scarring moxibustion,
— blistering moxibustion,
— scarring moxibustion.

### *Non-scarring moxibustion*

Place a medium or small-sized cone onto the selected area of skin and set light to it. Take it away, either before it has burnt down completely or before the patient starts to feel burning. Replace it with a new cone and set light to this. The skin should not be burned, nor should any blisters appear. With a medium-sized moxa, the patient will start to feel burning when $\frac{1}{4}$ or $\frac{2}{5}$ of the cone has been burned, at which point it should be taken away. With grain-sized cones, the cone should be crushed with a fingernail as soon as the patient feels pain, and then replaced with another to continue the moxibustion.

This technique of moxibustion is used to treat Empty or Cold diseases, for example lumbar pains, diarrhoea, abdominal pains, impotence, etc.

### *Blistering moxibustion*

For this type of moxibustion small-sized cones are used. Light the moxa and wait until the patient can feel burning, then leave the moxa to burn for another 3–5 seconds. A yellow ring may form on the skin, with a blister appearing after an hour or two. This should not be pierced, but covered with a dressing for protection, so that it can be resorbed on its own.

This kind of moxibustion is used in cases of asthma, tuberculosis and tuberculous lymph nodes.

### *Scarring moxibustion*

Before the treatment, place the patient in a comfortable position. He should not move from this position. Locate the selected points accurately and rub each one with a little garlic juice so that the moxa cone will stay in place. Light the cone and wait until it has burned down completely before replacing it with the next one. Continue with the moxibustion until the requisite number of cones for the treatment has been used.

The patient will usually feel extreme pain at the start of the moxibustion. Tapping the skin gently around the moxa cone will ease this. Intradermal anaesthetic may be injected into the points before treatment.

At the end of the moxibustion, the area treated will be burned, and may even look black. Clean it with a gauze compress and apply a little vaseline or ointment before covering (in China Qingshui ointment is used: 150–200 g of minium cooked in 500 g of sesame oil).

A week after moxibustion a whitish coloured non-bacterial discharge will appear at the points. The colour should be examined: if there is infection the discharge will be yellowy or greenish. Whilst the suppuration continues, renew the ointment and dressing every day. The site should scar over after 6 weeks.

If there is no discharge use a moxa stick over the point for 5–10 minutes once a day, for 2–3 days.

This technique, consisting as it does of burning, suppurating and scarring is used very little today. It does, however, give excellent results in the following cases:

— asthma: moxa Fengmeng BL 12, Feishu BL 13, Gaohuang BL 38, Shanzhong Ren 17,
— gastric or duodenal ulcers and oedema: moxa Shuifen Ren 9, Guanyuan Ren 4, Qihai Ren 6, Zusanli ST 36,
— impotence and reduced sexual potency in men: moxa Qihai Ren 6 and Zusanli ST 36,
— maintenance of health and as a preventative treatment: moxa Zusanli ST 36, Guahuang BL 38, and Qihai Ren 6.

### *Observations*

1. Accurate point location is very important. A divider or measuring string may be used to measure the distances, and the location of the point

should be marked with a dermagraphic pencil. The second phalanx of the left third finger for men, and of the right third finger for women is taken as a unit of measurement. If the treatment requires that the patient should be sitting up, locate the points when he is sitting; if the treatment requires that he lie down, locate the points when he is lying down.

2. The patient should be placed in a comfortable position so that he will not need to move.

3. The patient should be warned that he will feel heat and may experience pain. Note that women are better able to bear the pain than men.

4. To reduce the size of the scar the moxa can be moulded into a 'pip' shape, but this is unstable and the moxa may fall over.

5. Use an incense stick to light direct moxa. The right hand should be kept very steady when the moxa is small; maximum concentration is necessary when using 'pip'-shaped moxas.

6. The moxa is burnt from the top downwards. The pain is most intense when the cone turns white and looks like a ball of grey-white ash. This is the time to tap around the point to diminish the pain. To minimise pain, the first moxa should be very small. When it has burnt down, the skin will be dead and the sensations less intense. Generally, the progression in moxa size for men is: small, medium then large, and for women: small, small then medium.

7. When using non-scarring moxibustion, it may be necessary to increase the number of moxas to obtain a therapeutic effect.

8. When using several moxas in a row, remove the excess ash after the first one has burnt down, placing the next cone onto the ash which remains stuck to the skin, and continue in the same way.

9. When the moxibustion is finished and the wound has been dressed, the patient should avoid exercise and be careful not to catch a chill. In the days following treatment he should not shower and avoid wetting the places which have been treated. If a blister has formed, it should not be pierced.

10. Direct moxa quickens the pulse, stimulates the appetite, improves fitness, encourages sleep, and occasionally causes a temperature. Annual sessions of direct moxa should be enough for a 50-year-old man to maintain health and prevent weakening of Kidney Yang.

11. It is better not to use direct moxibustion during menstruation when treating women who have no menstrual disorders, or who are not being treated for problems of this type.

12. Direct moxa can be either reinforcing or reducing, but it is generally more reinforcing than reducing. Chapter 51 of the *Ling Shu* says that, to reinforce, the moxa should be left to burn slowly, and that, to reduce, the moxa should be fanned as soon as it is lit, so that it burns up quickly.

**Indirect moxibustion**

In indirect moxibustion, medicinal substances are placed in between the skin and the moxa cone. This is doubly effective. On the one hand, the action of the medication works in conjunction with that of the moxibustion; on the other hand, heat is released more evenly than in direct moxibustion. This technique is particularly suited to the treatment of chronic diseases and infections and ulceration of the skin.

Listed below are 11 variations of indirect moxibustion, although Wang Xue Tai of the Beijing Academy of Research into Traditional Medicine has described a total of 37.

### 1. Moxa with garlic (Allium sativum)

There are two different techniques: moxa on slices of garlic (Ge Suan Jiu) and moxa on garlic paste (Suan Ni Jiu).

*Garlic slices*

Take a clove of garlic and cut a slice 0.5–1 fen (3 mm) thick. Make several small holes in it and place it on the acupuncture point or the area to be treated. Put a small moxa cone on top of it and light it.

When the cone has completely burnt down, add another one and continue until the desired number of moxas have been used (generally between 3 and 6).

Replace the garlic if it dries out. By the time the moxibustion is completed, the skin should be red and slightly moist, and the patient should feel relaxed. There should be no pain or blistering.

*Action.* Cools Heat, dispels toxins, invigorates

the Blood, disperses masses, eases pain and dissipates swellings.

**Indications.** Boil, carbuncle, initial stage of pyogenic skin infections, insect and snake bite, incipient skin ulcer, osseous tuberculosis, tuberculous lymph nodes.

### Garlic paste

When the area to be treated is quite large, the garlic is made into a paste and put into a poultice. This should cover the whole area to be treated and be 3 mm thick. Make a few holes in the poultice, then place it in position. Use fairly large moxas. Continue with moxibustion until the poultice has dried out.

Garlic poultices can be prepared in advance, heat dried, then soaked in vinegar before use.

### 2. Moxa on chives (Jiu Cai Jiu) (Allium tuberosum).

This requires whole chives. The slices are taken from the bulb (the white part). The uses and indications are similar to moxa on garlic.

### 3. Moxa on aconite (Fu Zi Jiu)

The technique requires prepared root of aconite (prepared *Aconitum carmichaeli*). There are two different methods: aconite poultice and aconite root.

### Aconite poultice

Take some prepared aconite root and grind it into powder. Add a little water or white wine and make a 3 mm thick poultice to cover the area to be treated. Make a few holes in the poultice, then place it on the skin. Place a medium-sized moxa in position and light it. When the patient starts to feel pain from the burning take the moxa away and replace it. Continue moxibustion until the poultice dries out.

**Action.** Warms the Kidneys, strengthens original Yang (Kidney Yang), strengthens the holding function of Qi, arrests sweating, renews the flesh, purges impurities.

**Indications:**

— Internal medicine: Empty Kidney energy, impotence, premature ejaculation, Empty Yang and spontaneous sweating; collapse of Yang, heart failure; lower abdomen cold and painful; Emptiness and Cold in Spleen and Stomach; diarrhoea; Cold Bi.
— External medicine: chronic suppurating skin ulcer which will not scar over, fistula; very effective for speeding up scarring.

### Aconite slices

In cases of small incipient ulcers, the paste can be replaced with several 2–3 mm thick slices of prepared aconite root. Use small moxa cones. The technique is similar to moxa on slices of garlic.

### 4. Moxa on fresh ginger (Ge Jiang Jiu) (Rhizoma Zingiberis officinalis recens)

Cut a 5 mm thick slice of fresh ginger. Make several holes in it with a large needle and place it on the point or area to be treated. Place a moxa cone on top and light it (Fig. 6.3). When the patient feels a burning sensation remove the cone and replace it with another one. Continue until the slice of ginger dries out.

If the ginger dries out before the requisite number of cones have been burnt, put a fresh slice on top of the old one.

By the time the moxibustion is completed, the skin should be red and slightly moist and the patient should feel relaxed. There should be no pain or blistering.

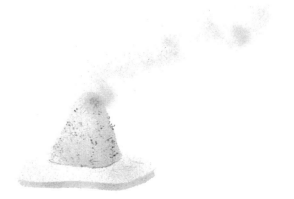

**Fig. 6.3** Indirect moxibustion on a slice of ginger.

*Indications:* Dyspepsia, abdominal pains, diarrhoea, spermatorrhoea, premature ejaculation, rheumatic pains (Feng Shi Bi) arising from Empty Cold.

## 5. *Moxa on white pepper* (Bai Hu Jiao Jiu)

Take a small quantity of white pepper, mix it with some flour and make a poultice 2 cm in diameter and 2 mm thick. Make a hollow in the centre of the poultice and fill it with a few pinches of powder composed of the following ingredients:

- *Syzygium aromaticum* (Ding Xiang): clove,
- *Moschus moschiferus* (She Xiang): musk,
- *Cortex cinnamomum* (Rou Gui): bark of cinnamomum cassia.

Place a moxa cone on the powder.
*Indications:* Wind, Cold and Damp Bi. Facial paralysis and paraesthesia.

## 6. *Moxa with fermented soya beans*

There are two variations:

— on its own,
— together with other medication.

*On its own*

Make a poultice with some fermented soya bean paste and place the moxa on top.
*Indications:* Boil, skin ulcer.

*Mixed with other medication*

Crush and mix the following ingredients:

- Fermented soya bean paste,
- *Zanthoxylum schinifolium,*
- *Rhizoma Zingiberis officinalis recens,*
- Sea salt,
- *Allium fistulosum* (the white part).

Use this paste to make a poultice 2 mm thick and 0.5–2 cm in diameter. Make a few holes in it, put a medium-sized moxa in position and light it.
*Indications:* Boil, carbuncle, initial stages of pyogenic skin infection.

## 7. *Moxa on loess* (Huang Tu Jiu)

Loess is a kind of very fine-grained chalky silt. Marl or very fine clay can be used in the same way.

Add water to a little purified clay to make a poultice 3 cm in diameter and 2 mm thick. Make a few holes in the poultice, place it in position and burn several large moxas in a row.
*Indications:* Boil and carbuncle, particularly on the back.

## 8. *Moxa on onion* (Ge Gong Jiu) (Allium fistulosum)

Place several slices of white onion on the patient's stomach, around the navel. Place large moxa cones on them and burn them at the same time or in sequence.
*Indications:* Shock, flatulence, Cold abdominal pains, anuria, urinary retention.

## 9. *Moxa on shallot* (Ge Xie Jiu) (Allium macrostemon chinense)

Preparation and indications are the same as for moxa on onion.

## 10. *Moxa pancake*

There are two techniques: 'flatiron' and 'solar'.
They are used for Empty Cold diseases, flaccid paralysis and Bi syndrome.

*'Flatiron' moxa* (Yun Jiu)

Distribute some moxa punk evenly over the point to be treated, cover it with several layers of cloth and place a hot iron on top. This technique combines the effect of mugwort with the heat of the flatiron.

*'Solar' moxa* (Ri Guang Jiu)

Place some moxa punk evenly on the patient's abdomen, then leave him in the sun for 10–20 minutes. This combines the effects of the mugwort with sunbathing and is particularly suitable for chronic constitutional weakness, changes in skin pigmentation and rickets in children.

### 11. Moxa on the navel

Numerous preparations can be used on the navel. Listed below are descriptions of three:

— moxa on sea salt,
— moxa on croton,
— moxa on medicinal powder.

#### Moxa on sea salt

Take enough sea salt to fill the navel. Heat it until any moisture had dried out, to prevent the grains from exploding under the heat of the moxa cone.

Place a gauze on the navel, fill it with the salt, put a large moxa on it and light. The number of moxas used depends on the disease and the condition of the patient.

**Actions:** Cools Heat, dispels toxins, strengthens the Stomach and the Intestines. Renews the Yang, treats Qi flowing the wrong way, strengthens the Lower Heater and the holding function of Qi to prevent leakages.

**Indications:** Acute gastroenteritis, intestinal disorders, vomiting, chronic diseases of the stomach and the intestines, anal prolapse, collapse from stroke (Zhong Feng).

**Observations:**

— In cases of empty Kidney Yang, manifesting itself as oedema, ascites, urinary retention or cardiac problems, different medicinal substances are added to the salt, for example (in ascending order of efficacy):
  • white pepper and a slice of ginger,
  • chives,
  • chives and musk,
  • chives, musk and a slice of ginger.
  (Make several holes in the ginger with a needle.)

— If the hollow in the navel is too small, make a crown around it out of paste (flour and water), clay or modelling clay.

— The moxa cone can be replaced by a piece of a large moxa stick (1 cm equals one cone). Make a hole in the centre of the cylinder of moxa, without pushing all the way through. The hole allows the smoke to descend so it is absorbed better. This method is recommended (Fig. 6.4).

— When menstruation is painful, moxa can be applied with the herb *Saussurea lappa*. It is impor-

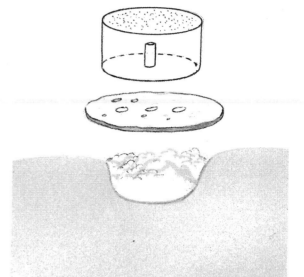

**Fig. 6.4** Moxa on the navel with salt, chives, musk and a slice of ginger. Replace the moxa cone with a piece of moxa stick: make a hole in the centre so that the smoke descends and is absorbed better.

tant to determine if the pain is Full or Empty. Premenstrual pain is generally considered to be a Full condition. These cases should be treated with needles. Postmenstrual pain usually arises from an Empty condition, and in these cases moxa can be used with confidence.

— If the patient feels a pronounced sensation of rising heat after moxibustion, burn a moxa on Zusanli ST 36 to rebalance the energy.

— After moxibustion, the practitioner may give the patient a glass of apple juice or cider.

#### Moxa on croton (Ba Dou Jiu) (Croton tiglium)

There are two techniques:

1. Take powdered rhizome of *Coptis chinensis* and 7 croton seeds which have been shelled without losing their oil, and crush them to a paste with a pestle and mortar. If the paste is too dry, too much Coptis powder has been used; add a few drops of water.

Put the paste onto the naval and burn moxas on it.

2. Take 10 croton seeds, crush, add 3 g of flour

and make up a paste. This is spread over the navel like a pancake. Burn 7 soya-bean-sized moxas, by which time there should be some intestinal borborygmus. Continue with moxa on onion (*Allium fistulosum*) or 'flatiron' moxa (see above). Finish by administering a decoction of:

- 3 g of powdered *Aconitum carmichaeli* (prepared),
- 1 slice of *Rhizoma Zingiberis officinalis recens*,
- 3 grains of sea salt,
- 6 g of Wu Ji powder (Wu Ji San).

This decoction is taken 3 times per day. It may induce slight perspiration.

*Formula for Wu Ji powder:*

| | |
|---|---|
| *Angelica sinensis* | |
| *Ligusticum Wallachii* | |
| *Paeonia alba* | 2.5 g each |
| *Poria cocos* | |
| *Platycodon grandiflorum* | |
| *Attractylodes sinensis* | |
| *Angelica dahurica* | 1.8 g each |
| *Magnolia officinalis* | |
| *Citrus reticulata* | |
| *Citrus aurantium* | 2.1 g |
| *Ephedra sinica* | |
| *Pinellia ternata* | 1.2 g each |
| *Cortex Cinnamomum cassia* | |
| *Rhizoma Zingiberis officinalis recens* | 0.9 g each |
| *Glycyrrhiza uralensis* | |

**Indications:** Dyspepsia, gastric pains from Cold, digestive problems.

*Medicinal moxa powder* (Zheng Qi Fa)

*Formula:*

| | |
|---|---|
| *Excrementum trogopterori* | 24 g |
| Sea salt | 15 g |
| *Boswellia carteris* | 3 g each |
| *Commiphora myrrha* | |
| *Vespertilio superans* (lightly grilled) | 6 g each |
| Dry *Allium fistulosum* | |
| *Akebia quinata* | 9 g |
| *Moschus moschiferus* | 0.2 g |

Grind all the ingredients into fine powder. Mix some of this with flour and water to make a small pancake, and place on the navel. The edges of the pancake should extend beyond the circumference of the navel. Put 6 g of the powder into the middle and cover it with a coin-sized sliver of *Sophora japonica* bark, then burn some moxas on it. Note the patient's age in years, and use the same number of moxas. Replenish the powder after each moxa.

**Indications:** Accumulation of Empty Cold, weak constitution; reinforces the Spleen and Stomach, increases resistance to infection, enhances the organism's prophylactic capabilities.

## MOXIBUSTION WITH A MOXA STICK

The use of moxa sticks, also known as moxa rolls or cigars, began during the Ming dynasty. The moxa stick evolved from medicinal sticks which were also known as fire arrows. This method of moxibustion uses two techniques: 'suspended cauterisation' (Xuan Qi Jiu) and 'cauterisation with pressure' (Shi'an Jiu).

'Suspended cauterisation' is usually administered with ordinary moxa sticks, whereas 'cauterisation with pressure' requires the use of medicinal sticks. Whichever technique is used, these procedures are all classified as indirect moxibustion.

### Making a moxa stick from mugwort

*Materials:*

- moxa punk
- a plywood box, 24 × 18 × 8 cm, light but strong
- strong brown wrapping paper
- a round hardwood baton, 34 cm long, 1.5 cm in diameter
- paper glue and wide adhesive tape, the strongest available.
- a sheet of cigarette paper measuring 18 × 8 cm (smaller cigarette papers can be stuck together to make up a large sheet). Rice paper can be used for want of anything better, but it gives off much more smoke.

*Preparation*

Cut a strip of wrapping paper 30 cm long and 18 cm wide. Place it on the box, matching the width of the paper to the width of the box. Position the paper so that there is an overhang of approximately 2 cm, then fold it over and attach it to the side of the box with the adhesive tape.

Wind the free end of the paper around the baton, keeping it well centred. After one or two turns make sure the paper is tightly wound and straight, then stick it down. The paper should be stuck to the wood first, then to itself. The stick should be rolled under the paper so that it ends up between the paper and the surface of the box. Leave it to dry for about an hour.

The assembly of stick and wrapping paper will be referred to as the handle of the apparatus.

### Making the moxa stick

Put some moxa punk next to the handle, along the entire width of the paper. Distribute it evenly as if making an old-fashioned roll-up cigarette. Lift the handle over the moxa and place it on the other side (Fig. 6.5a).

Hold the two ends of the handle and rotate it in the direction of the natural flow of the paper. Keep the paper taut and give the handle 2 or 3 turns so that the moxa is rolled and compressed (Fig. 6.5b). With the flat end of a pencil, tamp down each end of the newly formed roll.

Take the $18 \times 8$ cm roll of cigarette paper, place it under the handle and wind it in until only the free edge is showing. Apply glue to this or moisten it if it is already gummed.

Continue winding the handle in the same direction until the gummed paper has disappeared around the wad of moxa. Hold it in place for a few seconds then release the roll.

Apply glue to the outer edges of each end of the moxa stick and close them off, smoothing them down with your thumbnail. Brush the surface of the stick with egg white to keep the Qi of the mugwort inside.

### Moxibustion with medicated sticks

A little bit of musk (*Moschus moschiferus*) is generally put into all moxa sticks, but other substances can be used, for example the combination of:

*Cortex Cinnamomum cassia*
*Zingiber officinale* (dried)
*Flos Caryophilli*
*Saussurea lappa*
*Rhizoma Angelica pubescens*
*Radix Angelic dahurica*
*Rhizoma Atractylodes chinensis*
*Asarum sieboldii*
Realgar (see important note, p. 92)
*Boswellia carterii*
*Commiphora myrrha*
*Zanthoxylum piperitum.*

These medications are ground to a powder, then mixed in with the mugwort, 3 g per stick. The thickness of paper should be tripled.

Other substances can be added to the medicated sticks, for example:

*Aquilaria agallocha*
Sulphur
*Notopterygium incisium*
*Squama Manistis pentadactylae*
*Cortex Eucommia ulmoides*
*Citrus aurantium*

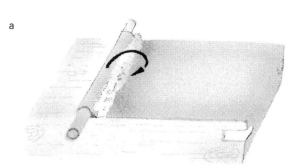
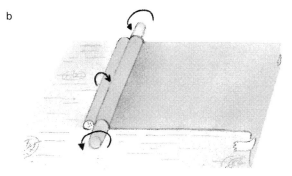

**Fig. 6.5a, b** Making a moxa stick. **a** Stage 1: put the moxa punk on the paper. **b** Stage 2: turn the handle to compress the moxa.

*Artemisia capillaris*
*Mylabris phalerata*
*Cortex Prunus persica*
*Radix Ligusticum wallichii*
*Buthus martensi*
*Croton tiglium*
*Gleditsia sinensis*
*Lignum Pini Nodi.*

### Suspended moxibustion (Xuan Qi Jiu)

An ordinary moxa stick is used, although occasionally a medicated stick may be appropriate. The practitioner lights the stick and holds it above the acupuncture point. The patient should be able to feel a sensation of heat, but the skin should never be burned. The procedure generally lasts 5–10 minutes.

#### Indications

Suspended moxibustion should be used in Stomach and Spleen syndromes of Emptiness and Cold, male impotence, dysentery, cystitis, and when the lower abdomen is painful and cold, as well as in rheumatoid arthritis, paraesthesia and paralysis.

#### Holding the moxa stick

a. The moxa stick is held like a pen between the thumb, index and third fingers. The little finger rests near the point being cauterised. This stops the wrist from shaking and prevents fatigue after lengthy moxibustion.

b. The moxa stick is held like a pen between thumb and index finger, and the third finger rests near the point.

#### Different moxibustion techniques

**Moxibustion with constant moderate heat (Wen He Jiu).** Bring the lighted end of the moxa stick near the point, roughly 1 or 2 cun above the skin. The patient should be able to feel a sensation of heat but not pain. The burning end of the moxa stick should be moved nearer or further away according to his reactions (Fig. 6.6).

Throughout the session, the distance should be adjusted according to the sensations felt by the patient. In general, the points are heated until the skin becomes red and congestive, but there should be no blistering.

The burning end should not be brought too close to the skin as the pain caused will necessitate stopping the moxibustion. As the aim is to heat the point, the procedure must continue for a while.

This technique clears the channels and collaterals (Jing Luo) and expels external Cold.

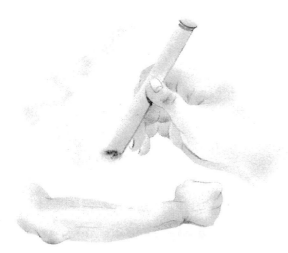

**Fig. 6.6** Holding the moxa stick: moxibustion with constant moderate heat.

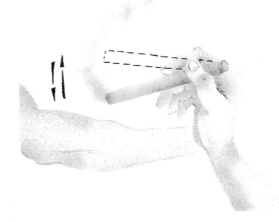

**Fig. 6.7** Holding the moxa stick: sparrow pecking moxibustion.

***Sparrow pecking moxibustion (Que Zhuo Jiu) also known as raising and lowering.*** Place the lighted end of the moxa stick over the point, about 2 cun away from the skin. Move the stick up and down, raising and lowering the burning end, like a sparrow pecking at grain (Fig. 6.7). The duration of the moxibustion should be monitored closely: this should rarely be more than 5 minutes, and generally should last 1 or 2 minutes. Care should be taken not to burn the skin by bringing the lighted end too close.

*Indications.* Loss of consciousness, syncope, Wind, Damp and Cold Bi.

***Ironing moxibustion (Yun Re Jiu).*** Place the lighted end of the moxa stick about 1 cun away from the skin. Move it backwards and forwards horizontally over the point as if ironing a shirt. The moxa stick should be parallel to the surface of the skin and the moxibustion should last 5–10 minutes.

*Indications:* Skin diseases, dermatosis, chilblains, Damp or Wind Bi affecting a large area, paralysis and paraesthesia.

### Recommendations

— Stop the moxibustion when the area has become congestive. Moxibustion can be applied to the same area once or twice daily.

— If the patient feels burning pain the treatment should be stopped, even if the point has not been warmed for the required amount of time. To maximise the diffusion of the heat avoid bringing the moxa stick too close to the skin.

— If it is necessary to make the heat penetrate deeply, use sparrow pecking moxibustion and press on the point with the left hand. This technique is very good for the relief of pain caused by Cold.

— If the area to be heated is quite large, circular ironing technique may be used, especially in skin diseases. Starting on the outer edges of the area, move the moxa stick round in smaller and smaller circles until it reaches the centre. Once there, lift the moxa stick up and start again on the outside. Moving the stick clockwise has no particular significance.

— In suspended moxibustion:
Reinforce by sparrow pecking, pressing on the point to make the heat penetrate. It is important to keep the fingers of your left hand close to the point to monitor the level of heat and prevent the skin being burned. Reduce by moving the stick in a circle at a constant distance from the point without pressing on it with your hand (Fig. 6.8).

### Personal techniques of suspended moxibustion

Always work with two moxa sticks at a time.

#### a. Reinforcing moxa on a specific point

Place your left hand flat on the skin, your third finger marking the point. Hold the two sticks in your right hand like two pencils, side by side, and bring the lighted ends to about 1 cm above the point, the hypothenar eminence of your right hand resting on the patient.

Leave the burning ends above the point for 1 second, then lift the sticks away quickly, pivoting your hand on the hypothenar eminence and keeping in contact with the patient's body. Leave the sticks in the air for 1 second, then bring them back over the point. Continue these movements rhythmically in sequence.

After three cauterisations cover the point with

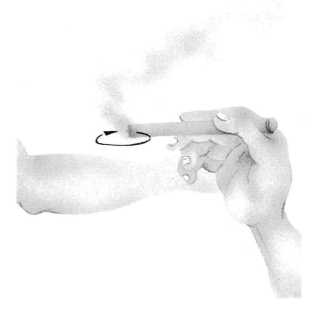

**Fig. 6.8** Reducing with suspended moxibustion.

the fingers of your left hand and allow it to cool for 2 or 3 seconds.

After 6 or 7 minutes this procedure will induce a penetrating sensation of heat, which may become difficult for the patient to bear. The procedure should therefore be terminated.

Heat the point until a red patch appears, but never till the skin is burnt. If this does happen, apply olive oil to the affected area.

#### b. Diffusing moxibustion

The area or points to be treated are heated by moving two sticks in a large circular movement.

Place your left hand flat on the skin near the area to be cauterised. Hold the moxa sticks in your right hand using the method described above for reinforcing, but without resting on the skin. Starting at the centre, heat the area or points with a large, circular movement.

This procedure induces a beneficial relaxing sensation in the area treated.

#### c. Cauterising the back Shu points

This technique makes it possible to treat the same two points on the inner Bladder lines on either side of the spine at the same time.

Hold the moxa sticks as if they were chopsticks, placing your third finger in between them, with the unlighted ends resting together on the metacarpo-phalangeal joint of your index finger. Cover the sticks and keep them in place with your thumb. The lighted ends are held apart from each other, and can cover both points to be treated.

Place the hypothenar eminence of your right hand on the patient's back, raising and lowering the sticks in the same way as for reinforcing moxibustion. Place your left hand flat on the patient's back, facing longitudinally along the dorsal spine, with the third finger in contact with the spinous processes of the vertebrae.

To cool the points down periodically, leave the third finger in place but flex it at the proximal interphalangeal joint so that it ends up resting on the posterior side of the distal phalanx. This movement brings the index and little fingers forwards, so that the fingertips can press the heated points for a few seconds. Put your hand back in position and continue with the moxibustion.

### Moxibustion with pressure (Shi'an Jiu)

This type of moxibustion is based on ancient techniques which comprise using mugwort moxa sticks together with medicinal powders. The two most commonly used preparations are miracle needle (Tai Yi Shen Zhen) and miracle thunderfire needle (Lei Huo Shen Zhen).

#### a. Miracle needle

*Medicinal powder ingredients:*

| | |
|---|---|
| Moxa punk | 100 g |
| Sulphur | 6 g |
| *Moschus moschiferus* | |
| *Boswellia carterii* | |
| *Commiphora myrrha* | |
| *Pinus massoniana* | |
| *Cinnamomum cassia* | |
| *Eucommia ulmoides* | |
| *Citrus aurantium* | |
| *Gleditsia sinensis* | 3 g each |
| *Asarum sieboldii* | |
| *Ligusticum wallachii* | |
| Realgar (see important note, p. 92) | |
| *Manis pentadactyla* | |
| *Angelica dahurica* | |
| *Buthus martensii* | |

Grind these ingredients to a fine powder and mix well.

**Making the moxa stick.** Take a sheet of fairly strong paper (Sang Pi Zhi mulberry bark paper), and distribute 25 g of moxa punk evenly over it. Add 6 g of the medicinal powder, and mix it in well with the moxa punk. Roll up the moxa stick, coat the outside with egg white, and stick another sheet of mulberry paper around it. Leave 1 cun of excess paper at either end and close them off with a twist.

**Application.** There are two techniques:

a. Steam some non-synthetic cloth over a decoction of the above preparation, then wrap several layers around the lighted end of the moxa stick. Place the moxa on the point, relighting if it goes out and cools down. The moxa stick may be relit 5–7 times. Press it down hard on the point until the patient can feel the heat. Lift the stick away as soon as he feels burning, then start again.

b. Steam some non-synthetic cloth over a decoction of the above preparation, then place several layers on the points to be treated. Put the burning end of the moxa stick onto the cloth over the point, leaving it there for 1 or 2 seconds, then move it to another point. The moxa should be placed on each point a dozen times.

'Miracle needle' is considered to be very effective in the treatment of Wind, Cold and Damp Bi, flaccid paralysis, and Empty-Cold syndromes, especially in those causing dysmenorrhoea and abdominal pain.

### b. Miracle thunder-fire needle

*Ingredients:*

| | |
|---|---|
| *Moxa punk* | 60 g |
| *Aquilaria agallocha* | |
| *Saussurea lappa* | |
| *Boswellia carterii* | |
| *Artemisia capillaris* | 10 g each |
| *Notopterigium incisum* | |
| *Zingiber officinale* (dried) | |
| *Manis pentadactyla* | |
| *Moschus moschiferus* | 0.5 g |

The preparation, application and indications of this compound are the same as for the miracle needle.

## FUMIGATION WITH MOXA (Ai Xun Jiu)

Fumigation is a procedure using the therapeutic properties of smoke or steam derived from medicinal compounds. There are several fumigation techniques:

***Fumigation with steam:*** Boil some mugwort in water. Use the steam from the boiling water for fumigation, either with the water still boiling or, when the decoction is completed, by pouring the boiling water into a bowl.

***Fumigation by 'moxa box'.*** A smoke machine is used. There are several types, usually made from a perforated cylindrical tube of metal. The moxa punk is burned inside the tube and the points are fumigated with the hot smoke escaping from the holes.

***Fumigation with a glass.*** Put some moxa punk in a glass and set light to it, and use the smoke to fumigate the selected points.

***Fumigation with a moxa stick.*** This is a technique frequently used by us, and is derived from our method of burning moxas on salt on the navel. Take a piece of moxa stick 1 cun long and make a hole in the centre. Light one of the ends and bring the unlit end to the point. The smoke will escape from the hole in the centre and impregnate the point.

Whichever fumigation technique with mugwort is used, the treated area should not be cleaned afterwards.

***Associated diseases:*** Bi syndrome, abdominal distension, diarrhoea, chronic Cold type abdominal pains.

## B. MOXA WITHOUT MUGWORT

There are numerous other products which can be used for moxibustion but generally they are used for supplementary techniques. There are many such techniques, and only the main ones are mentioned here:

### Moxa with sulphur

Indications: abscess, boil, fistula.

Take a piece of sulphur, roughly the same size as the boil. Place the sulphur on the boil and light it with another piece of sulphur, which should already be lit.

### Moxa with wax

Indications: ulcer, boil, carbuncle.

Make a paste from flour and water, and shape it into a crown about 1 cun high around the ulcer or boil. Put several strips of wax inside the crown. Melt the wax with a live coal which is withdrawn as soon as the patient feels the heat. In cases of deep and extensive ulceration, the patient will not feel any pain, and more wax should be added as necessary. As soon as the patient begins to feel local irritation the procedure should be stopped and a few drops of cold water should be poured onto the wax. When it has cooled, both wax and paste should be removed.

### Moxa with tobacco

Indications: Warms the vessels and disperses cold. In emergencies cigarettes can be used instead of moxa sticks. Care should be taken, as they burn less evenly and at a higher temperature than mugwort.

### Moxa with mulberry or peach wood

Indications: rheumatism, abscess, boil, ulcer, tuberculous lymph nodes.

Take a dry twig of mulberry or peach and light one end. Blow on it to put out the flame and apply moxibustion with the glowing tip. The skin should not be burned, but the patient should be able to feel some irritation of the area treated.

### Moxibustion with rush pith

The name is derived from the use of rush pith soaked in oil as a wick for a lamp. The technique is also known as moxibustion with lamp wick.

Take some rush pith soaked in sesame oil and light it. Use the lighted end to apply moxibustion to the points to be treated by touching the wick to the skin and quickly pulling it away. The skin should not be burned. This technique disperses Wind, clears the surface, opens the chest, moves Qi, clears Phlegm, calms the spirit (Shen) and eases spasms.

*Indications.* This is a common technique to treat pains in the stomach and abdomen, malaria, parotitis, indigestion in children and infantile convulsions.

## MOXA WITHOUT HEAT

This moxa effect is not accomplished through the application of heat but through the vesicatory action of the products used.

### Moxa with garlic paste

Take some garlic, preferably purple-skinned, and crush it into a paste. Put this in a poultice on the point to be treated:

- Hegu LI 4: treats tonsillitis.
- Yuji LU 10: indicated in pharyngitis.

### Moxa with Evodia rutaecarpa *paste*

Grind some Evodia fruits into powder. Mix this powder with a little vinegar to make a poultice, and place it on Yongquan KI 1. Replace the poultice once a day.

*Indications:* oedema in children.

### Moxa with Ranunculus japonicus *leaf paste (buttercup)*

Crush some buttercup leaves and make up a paste. When the poultice is placed on the points it causes irritation with congestion and blistering.

*Indications:*

- Malaria: Jingqu LU 8, Neiguan P 6, Dazhui Du 14.

### Moxa with Eclipta prostrata *paste*

Crush into a paste and apply to the points in a poultice until a blister appears.

Example: Dazhui Du 14 for malaria.

### Moxa with Rhizoma Euphorbiae kansui *paste*

Grind the rhizome to a fine powder, then apply in a poultice to Dazhui Du 14 to treat malaria.

### Moxa with Ricinus communis *paste*

Take some shelled castor oil plant seeds and crush them to make a paste.

- A poultice on Baihui Du 20 treats uterine prolapse.
- A poultice on Yongquan KI 1 eases labour in difficult delivery.

### Moxa with white mustard seed paste

Powdered white mustard mixed with water is

effective against rheumatic pains when applied in a poultice.

*Powder:*

| | |
|---|---|
| *Corydalis Turtschaninovii* | 30 g |
| *Euphorbia kansui* | 30 g |
| *Asarum sieboldii* | 30 g |
| *Moschus moschiferus* | 1.5 g |

Grind these ingredients to a powder, and mix with white mustard powder and water to make a paste.

Poultices on Feishu BL 13, Gaohuang BL 38, Bailao (extra point) are indicated for asthma. When the poultice is in place it will produce smarting sensations and pain but these will disappear after an hour or two. Change the poultice once a day. The course of treatment should last for about 10 days.

### Cold moxa on the navel

Put a compress on the navel and fill the umbilical cavity with alum powder. Pour cold water onto the alum, one drop at a time. A sensation of cold will penetrate into the abdomen, easing urination and bowel motion. This technique is indicated in Heat syndromes with anuria and constipation.

If the navel is not very deep, make a crown around it out of paste (flour and water) or modelling clay, as described above in the section on moxas on the navel.

## PRINCIPLES FOR TREATMENT WITH MOXIBUSTION

### Indications

*1. Heats to disperse Perverse energy: Wind, Cold and Damp*

Through its heating action moxibustion can re-establish a fluid circulation of Qi and Blood, relaxing the muscles and tendons and strengthening the functional activity of the digestive tract.

It is therefore used to treat:

- Wind, Cold and Damp Bi,
- abdominal pain, gastrointestinal problems, diarrhoea and dysmenorrhoea arising from Cold.

*2. Heats to benefit the circulation in the Channels and Collaterals*

The properties of moxibustion are used to heat the channels, regulating the circulation of Qi and Blood, stopping pain arising from stagnation of Qi or Accumulation of Blood.

It is therefore used to treat:

- paraesthesia, pain, dysmenorrhoea, and swellings caused by stagnation of Qi and Accumulation of Blood, either localised or blocking a channel or collateral.

*3. Increases Qi and nourishes the Blood*

Moxibustion is used to treat weakness of the organism in chronic disease:

- muscular atrophy, paralysis, chronic diarrhoea, chronic cystitis, chronic nephritis, malposition of the fetus and agalactia from deficiency of the organism.

*4. Warms the Kidneys, strengthens Kidney Yang, tonifies central Qi and stops prolapse and bleeding*

Moxibustion is used to treat:

- impotence, spermatorrhoea, premature ejaculation, diseases arising from Emptiness and Cold in the Stomach, gastric and uterine prolapse and chronic enteritis.

*5. Renews the Yang, treats collapse of Yang*

This is why moxibustion is used to treat loss of consciousness with shortness of breath, weak pulse, closed eyes, with or without spasms in the limbs.

*6. Clears and dissipates toxic Heat*

Moxibustion is used for its analgesic, scarring and dissipatory action in pyogenic infections, and dissolves clots and 'accumulations'. It is used to treat:

- boil, carbuncle, mastitis, snakebite, scorpion sting, pulmonary or lymphatic tuberculosis, hernia pains (Shan Qi), fistula and ulcers which will not scar over.

## 7. Prophylaxis

Textbooks frequently mention the preventative properties of moxibustion. For example:

- The *Yishuo* recommends moxa on Zusanli ST 36 to protect against stroke (Zhong Feng).
- Zhang Gaozhuan (1224) writes that moxa on Zusanli ST 36 increases health and that moxa on Guanyuan Ren 4 and on Shenshu BL 23 strengthens original Yang.
- It is common knowledge that moxa on Dazhui Du 14, Fengmen BL 12, Hegu LI 4 can protect against Gan Mao (acute upper respiratory tract infection, e.g. flu, etc.).

It should, however, be remembered that this preventative effect depends on the correct use of the moxas, and in particular on the use of blistering direct moxibustion. This is stated by Yang Jizhou in scroll 9 (Quian Jin Jiu Fa) of the *Zhen Jiu Da Cheng* (1601): 'If it is necessary to strengthen the person's good health, Zusanli ST 36 should never be dry'. This means that direct moxibustion should cause non-bacterial suppuration at Zusanli.

## Contraindications

There are several contraindications for moxibustion:

- febrile diseases, rapid pulse and Empty Yin,
- cases of empty Yin and internal Heat (Empty Heat), as moxibustion may increase the Fire and disturb the 'pure openings',
- full Heat syndromes,
- headache from excess Liver Yang,
- spastic stroke (closed Zhong Feng),
- in cases of malnutrition, or if the patient's constitution is too weak, if the patient has had too much to eat, or if he is drunk.

— Be extremely cautious in cases of loss of fluid, profuse sweating, loss of blood and generalised oedema.

— Avoid moxibustion on the points of the lower abdomen and the lumbo-sacral area on pregnant women.

— Do not apply direct moxa to the face, or close to the orifices of the body, to areas which are very hairy, to scars, to places where the person is very emaciated, and to the joints of the wrist and ankle.

— Do not perform moxa around the heart area, around the eyes, on the neck or the nape of the neck, on the sexual organs, or near a mucous membrane or a major blood vessel.

### Points forbidden to moxa

This list of 43 points is taken from the 'litany of points forbidden to moxa' in the *Zhen Jiu Da Cheng*:

| | |
|---|---|
| Yamen Du 15 | Fengfu Du 16 |
| Tianzhu BL 10 | Chengguang BL 6 |
| Toulingqi GB 15 | Touwei ST 8 |
| Sizhukong TB 23 | Zanzhu BL 2 |
| Jingming BL 1 | Suliao Du 25 |
| Heliao LI 19 | Yingxiang LI 20 |
| Quanliao SI 18 | Xiaguan ST 7 |
| Renying ST 9 | Tianrong SI 17 |
| Tianfu LU 3 | Zhourong SP 20 |
| Jiuwei Ren 15 | Fuai SP 16 |
| Jianzhen SI 9 | Yangchi TB 4 |
| Zhongchong P 9 | Shaoshang LU 11 |
| Yuji LU 10 | Jingqu LU 8 |
| Diwuhui GB 42 | Yaoyangguan Du 3 |
| Jizhong Du 6 | Yinbai SP 1 |
| Lougu SP 7 | Yinlingquan SP 9 |
| Tiakou ST 38 | Dubi ST 35 |
| Yinshi ST 33 | Futu ST 32 |
| Biguan ST 31 | Shenmai BL 62 |
| Weizhong BL 54 | Yinmen BL 51 |
| Chengfu BL 50 | Baihuanshu BL 30 |
| Xinshu BL 15 | |

Points on the face should be avoided, as moxibustion could cause suppuration and scarring. Renying and Weizhong are forbidden because they are near a major blood vessel. There are points on this list, however, which are quite beneficial when used with moxibustion. Yinbai SP 1 treats uterine bleeding (Benglou) and Dubi ST 35 is used for articular pains in the knee. Clinical experience has shown that in certain cases the ancient texts can be updated.

## Observations on the practice of moxibustion

1. Before a patient is treated with moxibustion he should be mentally prepared to accept that the heat may be painful.

2. The patient should be put in as comfortable a position as possible so that he can remain there without moving for the duration of the treatment.

3. The same points are used in moxibustion as in acupuncture, but the advantage of moxibustion is that it induces a sensation of relaxation and well-being in the patient.

4. The action of direct moxa is immediate and the therapeutic effect lasts for a long time, whereas with indirect moxa, especially when applied with a moxa stick, the effect is slower to take hold and of shorter duration.

5. If points on the legs and the arms are to be used, moxa should be administered to the arms first. The thorax and abdomen should be treated before the back and lumbar area.

6. The length of moxibustion and the number of moxas used should be greater on the lumbar region, the back and the abdomen than on the thorax and the limbs. The number of moxas should be even less on the head and neck.

7. If needling and moxibustion are going to be used together on a point, the needle should be inserted and manipulated first. When the needle has been withdrawn, moxibustion can be commenced. Another technique is to insert and manipulate the needle, then burn some moxa on it before withdrawing it (see below, 'Warm needle', Ch. 7).

8. If the onset of the disease is recent and the organism is still strong, moxas should be applied liberally to begin with and the number reduced as the patient gets better. In chronic disease when the organism has become weak the number of moxas should be reduced at the start and increased as the disease improves.

9. If the patient is young more moxas can be used, but the number should be reduced for elderly people and children. The number of moxas should be increased in Empty syndromes, Cold syndromes, in winter, and in regions with a cold climate.

### Effects of moxibustion

Moxibustion tends to mobilise Qi rapidly.

— In collapse of Yang, with trembling, sweating and dizziness, moxa on Qihai Ren 6 or Guanyuan Ren 4 restores the energy to the Centre.

— In Empty Fire rising upwards, moxa on Qihai Ren 6, Guanyuan Ren 4 or on the legs pulls down the Yang.

— In cases of arterial hypertension, moxa on Zusanli ST 36 or Fenglong ST 40 reduces arterial blood pressure.

— In dizziness arising from Emptiness in the head, moxa may be applied to Baihui Du 20. However, if the dizziness arises from Wind or Fullness it is possible that moxa on Baihui will aggravate the symptoms and provoke fever and headache. If this happens it is imperative to rebalance the energy by applying moxa to points on the lower part of the body.

— Moxa on the navel is very effective to tonify Qi, but misuse may lead to difficulties in sleeping. Great care should be taken when treating young people. Patients over 40 can have one treatment a year, and patients over 50 can have two.

Moxa on the navel makes energy rise to the upper part of the body. If the patient has a constitutional tendency for energy to rise, it may be aggravated by the moxa, especially when points higher up on the body are selected. To avoid this risk points low down on the body may be heated, e.g. Taixi KI 3, Fuliu KI 9, Yingu KI 10.

When points below the navel are used, the lower part of the body should be rebalanced. In this case the points mentioned above should only be needled.

After moxibustion the patient should not drink too much, and should avoid raw fruit and vegetables, fatty foods and alcohol. He should also abstain from sexual intercourse, remain calm and avoid getting cold.

**Important note**

In 1991 the British Council for Acupuncture alerted members to the possible risks of using realgar in moxibustion, as it gives off poisonous arsenic sulphide gas when burned. To avoid any chance of arsenic poisoning practitioners have been cautioned against the use of moxa sticks containing realgar until more information is made available. When making their own moxa sticks or cones readers are advised to omit realgar from the ingredients.

# 7. Other needle techniques

## CUTANEOUS NEEDLE (Pi Fu Zhen)

Treatment with a cutaneous needle (Pi Fu Zhen) consists of tapping the skin lightly with a group of needles. This technique is also known as 'skin pricking' because the stimulation is confined to the skin. It has been developed from the ancient techniques and types of needle discussed in Chapter 7 of the *Ling Shu* (Mao Ci, Ban Ci, Fu Ci), which consist of stimulating the skin with a short filiform needle.[1] The needle used today is descended from the arrow-shaped (Chan) and fine (Hao) needles described in Chapter 1 of the *Ling Shu* (see above, Ch. 1).

Cutaneous needling is not confined to local acupuncture points or painful areas on the body; it can be applied anywhere which is indicated by an overall understanding of Chinese medicine. Chapter 56 of the *Su Wen* says: 'Each of the 12 channels is located in a section of the skin, which is why disease first starts in the skin'. The 12 regions of the skin (Pibu) are closely linked to the 12 channels (Jingluo) and the 12 organs (Zangfu). Needling and tapping these regions enables Qi to flow from the organs to the channels (Shu Tong Jing Luo Zang Fu Zhi Qi), drains the channels and collaterals (Shu Tong Jing Luo) and regulates Qi and Blood, all of which rebalance the organism.

### Equipment

There are two kinds of cutaneous needle available: hammer-shaped and rolling drum.

### *Hammer-shaped needle*

This looks like a light hammer, with a long handle and a head dotted with small spines (Fig. 7.1). The classical hammer has a 30 cm handle which is round, strong and flexible. The modern hammer is made of plastic. The handle is also flexible, but shorter, and flattened at its free end. Short filiform needles are embedded in the head of the hammer in varying numbers: 5 for plum blossom needles (Mei Hua Zhen), 7 for 7 star needles (Qi Xing Zhen) and 18 for Arhat needles (Luo Han Zhen).[2]

The spines are shaped like pine needles. To check their condition bring them gently in contact with a piece of cotton wool; the cotton wool fibres will stick to any points which are defective. It is therefore a simple matter to identify and discard cutaneous needles with blunt, sharp, bent or missing spines.

When treating children and people with a very weak constitution, the hammer-shaped cutaneous needle can be replaced with a hard toothbrush. The corners of the bristles should be chamfered.

### *Rolling drum* (Gun Ci Tong)

This is a metal roller dotted with spines. It has the advantage of having a wide surface and can stimulate a large area of skin evenly. It is easy to handle.

### *Method*

The cutaneous needle has many advantages: it is

---

[1] Mao Ci — needle 'like a hair'; Ban Ci — half needling; Fu Ci - superficial needling.

[2] The Arhat (Sanskrit), Arahat (Pali) or Luo Han (Chinese) — disciples of Buddha grouped in numbers of 16, 18... 500.

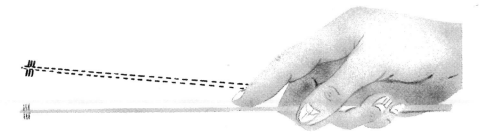

**Fig. 7.1**   Hammer-shaped cutaneous needle.

safe, effective, easy to handle and treats a broad range of conditions.

The instrument should be sterilised and the area to be treated disinfected with 75% alcohol.

*Hammer-shaped needle*

The classical hammer is held by the handle in the right hand, which is almost fully pronated:

— Hold the handle in place on the hypothenar eminence with your fourth and fifth fingers.
— Grip the top and the bottom of the handle with your thumb and index fingers.
— Extend your index finger and press down on the handle.
— The end of the handle should extend a few centimetres past the palm of your hand.

The modern hammer, which has a shorter handle flattened at the end, is held slightly differently. Position the thumb, index and third fingers as above, but press the handle into the palm of your hand with your fourth and fifth fingers. The handle should not stick out.

With the movement coming from the wrist, raise and lower the cutaneous needle regularly and smoothly, lifting it as soon as it makes contact with the skin. The spines should make contact at right angles (90°) to the surface of the skin, as any other angle of impact will cause intense pain.

The strength of tapping gives two principal types of stimulation:

— Gentle tapping, with very brief contact between needle and skin, produces gentle stimulation with slight reddening of the skin. This is reinforcing.
— Tapping and pressing, with longer contact between needle and skin, produces strong stimu-

lation with intense reddening of the skin, even a little bleeding. This is reducing.

Reinforcing is indicated for the elderly and patients with weak constitutions, chronic disease and symptoms of Emptiness. Reducing is indicated for young people, patients with strong constitutions, acute disease and symptoms of Fullness.

*Rolling drum*

Hold the handle in your right hand and roll the drum backwards and forwards over the skin. For gentle stimulation keep the handle parallel to the surface of the skin; for strong stimulation hold it at an angle of at least 45° to the skin.

**Locations to stimulate**

The places to stimulate follow the pathway of a channel, or extend around nerves or muscles. Tap from top to bottom and from the interior towards the exterior.

According to the condition of the disease, the technique consists of stimulating:

- an acupuncture point: selective tapping,
- a channel: linear tapping,
- a diseased area: area tapping, performed from the edges towards the centre.

These three techniques can be used on their own or in combination.

1. For diseases of the organs, treatment should start with 'primary tapping'. Whatever the disease, this technique consists of tapping along the inner Bladder line on either side of the spine, starting from the shoulders and moving to the lumbosacral area. This is done downwards and upwards

three times. There should be about 0.5–1 cun between each point of impact.

After primary tapping, points are chosen according to which organ is implicated in the disease.
Examples:

- Diseases of the respiratory system: apply stimulation between the 1st and 7th thoracic vertebrae (T1–T7),
- Diseases of the nervous system and psychological diseases: apply stimulation to T3 and L2 as well as the head,
- Diseases of the digestive system: apply stimulation between T7 and L5,
- Diseases of the genitourinary system: apply stimulation between L5 and the sacral vertebrae.

2. In diseases of the limbs and the skin 'primary tapping' may be omitted. Tap over the diseased area or follow the channel pathway.

***Tapping lines and indications*** (Figs. 7.2a, b and 7.3a, b)

### Back

Tap over the inner and outer Bladder lines, on both sides of the spine.

### Shoulder

Tap 3 or 4 lines outwards following the lower fibres of trapezius.

Indications: pain in the shoulder region, paralysis of the upper limb, diseases of the respiratory organs.

### Scapula

Tap 3 or 4 lines going upwards and outwards over the scapula.

Indications: pains in the scapula.

### Lumbar region

Tap 3 or 4 lines parallel to the spine, with a gap of 1 cm between each line.

Indications: lumbar pain, paralysis of the lower limb, diseases of the liver, gall bladder, pancreas, stomach and kidneys.

### Sacrum and buttocks

Tap 2 or 3 lines in an arc starting at the sacrum and going downwards and outwards over the buttocks.

Indications: lumbar pain, paralysis of the lower limb, urinary, genital and intestinal disease.

### Chest

*Sternum.* Tap 2 lines going downwards along the edges of the sternum.

*Sides.* Tap inwards along the intercostal spaces.

Indications: thoracic diseases, diseases of the heart and lungs.

### Abdomen

*Upper abdomen.* Tap 5–7 horizontal lines across the abdomen from the costal margin as far as the navel, then tap vertically downwards over the same area. Alternatively tap 3–5 lines following a series of arcs going outwards and downwards, parallel to the costal margin.

Indications: diseases of the liver, gall bladder, spleen and stomach.

*Lower abdomen.* Tap 5 vertical lines over the area from the navel to the pubis and above the groin, then go over the same area with 5 horizontal lines.

Indications: diseases of the reproductive organs.

### Head

*Top of the cranium (vertex) and forehead.* Tap 4–8 lines running parallel to the hairline, covering the area from the upper border of the eyebrows to the vertex. The direction of tapping is of no significance.

Indications: headache, neurasthenia.

*Occiput.* Tap 3 lines following the Du Mai, Bladder and Gall Bladder channels, covering the area from the occipital bone to Naohu Du 17, Yuzhen BL 9 and Fenchi GB 20.

Indications: headache, neurasthenia.

*Temples.* Tap 3–5 lines fanning out from the ears to the temples.

Indications: headache, neurasthenia.

a

b

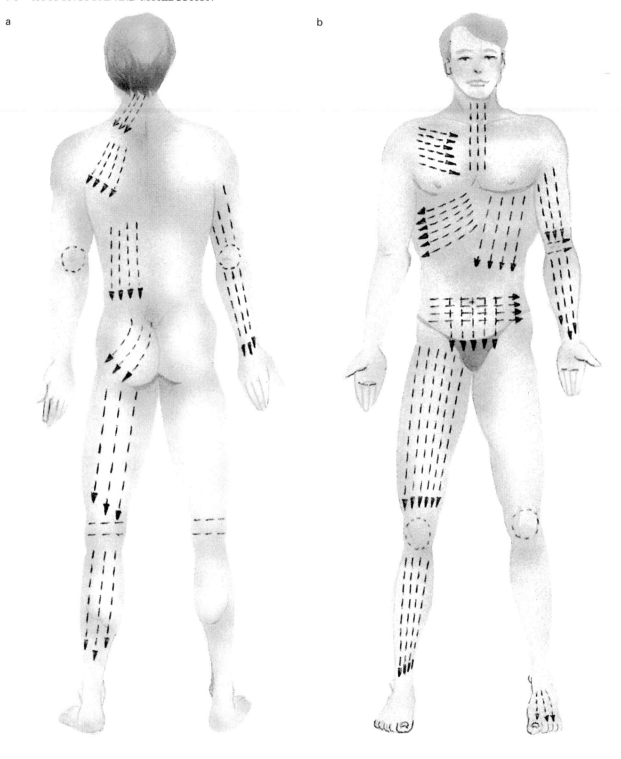

**Fig. 7.2a, b**    Tapping lines. **a** Body and limbs: Yang aspect. **b** Body and limbs: Yin aspect.

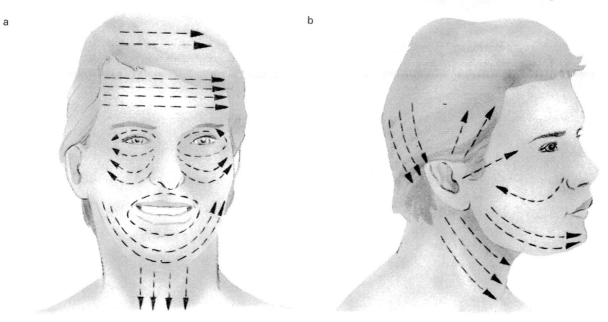

**Fig. 7.3a, b** Tapping lines. **a** Head: anterior aspect **b** Head: lateral aspect.

## Face

*Eyes.* Tap 4 horizontal lines outwards, keeping parallel to the upper and lower eyelids, or tap 1 or 2 curving lines around the orbit.

Indications: eye diseases, facial paralysis.

*Mouth.* Tap 1 or 2 lines following the curve of the lips.

Indications: facial paralysis.

*Lower jaw.* Tap 1 or 2 lines in an arc, following the line of the lower jaw. The direction of tapping is of no significance.

Indications: facial paralysis.

*Cheek.* Tap 3 lines going outwards following the curve of the zygomatic arch.

Indications: facial paralysis.

## Neck

Indications: neck diseases, diseases of the digestive system.

*Anterior neck.* Tap 1–3 lines running parallel to the anterior midline of the cranium.

*Lateral neck.* Tap 1–3 lines running parallel to sternocleidomastoid.

*Posterior neck.*

1. Tap 1 line running down the centre of the posterior neck from Naohu Du 17 to Dazhui Du 14.

2. Tap 2 lines down both sides of the posterior neck from Fengchi GB 20 and Tianzhu BL 10 to the transverse spines of C6.

3. Tap 3 lines running parallel to trapezius, from the upper medial area to the lower lateral area of the neck.

## Limbs

Follow the pathway of the 12 channels. Tap 1–2 lines for each channel. Circular tapping may be performed around the elbow, patella and the internal and external malleoli.

These general rules apart, the tapping lines can be modified according to the disease. The Ashi points corresponding to the location of the disease can be treated; for example, in circular baldness, tap in a circle following the edges of the bald patch.

## General indications

The cutaneous needle is particularly suitable for women, children and sensitive or elderly people. It can be used to treat headache, dizziness, insomnia, neurasthenia, chronic dermatosis, gastroenteritis, infantile paralysis, thoracic pain and chronic gynaecological disease.

## Examples

Please note for the purpose of the next series of examples the word 'point' denotes an area, a site or an area around the acupuncture point, and the terms 'needling' and 'tapping' are synonymous.

### Headache and migraine

For headache, the principal sites of treatment are the occiput and the cranium. Use points on the occiput or posterior neck and on the site of the pain, as well as distal or tender points on the pathways of the affected channels.

For migraine, use points on the posterior neck, on the side of the head where the pain is, and tender points on the pathway of the affected channels.

### Thoracic and costal pain

Principal sites: both sides of the spine level with T1–T12, especially over the points Geshu BL 17 and Ganshu BL 18.

Thoracic pain: needle the painful area, as well as above, below and to the sides of the pain.

Costal pain: add the points Zhigou TB 6 and Taichong LIV 3 to the above points.

### Insomnia

Principal sites: both sides of the spine, especially over the points Xinshu BL 15, Ganshu BL 18 and on the Heart and Pericardium channels.

In cases of insomnia with frequent dreaming and palpitations, add Fengchi GB 20, Sanyinjiao SP 6 or tender sites near these points.

In cases of somnolence, add sensitive sites on Du Mai and Ren Mai.

### Pain in the upper or lower limb, lumbar sprain

Principal sites:

Upper limb: both sides of the thoracic spine, the site of pain and tender points of Du Mai.

Lower limb: both sides of the lumbar spine, the site of pain on the upper and lower limb.

Lumbar sprain: the lumbar region, coccyx, tender places on both sides, and along the Bladder channel pathway on the lower limb.

### Facial paralysis

Principal sites: the affected part of the face and the points Zanzhu BL 2, Tongziliao GB 1, Dicang ST 4, Jiache ST 6 as the main points, and associated points Hegu LI 4, or tender points.

### Bi Zheng: numbness and/or stagnation of Qi/Xue, rheumatism.

Principal sites:

Pain in the upper limb: both sides of the thoracic spine and the shoulder and elbow joint.

Pain in the lower limb: both sides of the lumbar spine and the sites of pain. If the Bi Zheng is red and swollen (tumefied), strong needling with bleeding may be applied. If the site of the Bi Zheng is swollen, needle till the area is dotted with holes (dianci) and finish with cupping.

### Hiccough

Principal sites: T9–T12 and the midline of the abdomen, i.e. Ren Mai. The points Geshu BL 17, Ganshu BL 18, Weishu BL 21 and Tianshu ST 25, Daheng Sp 15 on the abdomen may be added.

### Wei Zheng (flaccid paralysis)

Principal sites:

Upper limb: both sides of the spine from T1–T7.

Lower limb: both sides of the lumbar and sacral spine.

If the upper limb is paralysed (Mabi), the 3 arm Yin and the 3 arm Yang channels may be added. If the lower limb is paralysed (Mabi) the pathways of the 3 leg Yin and the 3 leg Yang channels may be needled. Strong needling may be applied to the places where the joints are deformed.

### Gastric pain and vomiting

Principal sites: Ganshu BL 18, Pishu BL 20, Weishu BL 21, Zhongwan Ren 12. For gastric pain Gongsun SP 4, Zusanli ST 36 and local tender spots may be added. For vomiting, add strong needling to Neiguan P 6.

*Abdominal pain*

Principal sites: both sides of the spine from T9–L5, and on the abdomen.

If the pain is in the upper abdomen, add Shangwan Ren 13, Zhongwan Ren 12 and Youmen KI 21.

If the pain is in the lower abdomen, add Guanyuan Ren 4 and Qihai Ren 6.

*Asthma* (Xiaochuan), *cough* (Kesou)

Principal sites: both sides of the thoracic spine, points Feishu BL 13, Shanzhong Ren 17.

For asthma add Tiantu Ren 22, Tianshu ST 25.
For cough add Chize LU 5.
If there is phlegm (Tan), add Fenglong ST 40, or a tender point close to it.

*Urinary incontinence*

Principal sites: both sides of the lumbar and sacral spine, and the lower abdomen.

Add Sanyinjiao SP 6, Qihai Ren 6 for urinary incontinence in children.

Add Qihai Ren 6, Guanyuan Ren 4, Dahe Ren 12 for adults.

*Spermatorrhoea and impotence*

Principal sites: both sides of the lumbar and sacral spine, and the midline of the abdomen, on Ren Mai.

For spermatorrhoea add Guanyuan Ren 4.
For impotence add Ciliao BL 32, Dahe KI 12.
If the patient suffers from disturbed sleep add Sanyinjiao SP 6.

*Palpitations*

Principal sites: Xinshu BL 15, Ganshu BL 18.

Add Shenmen HT 7, Sanyinjiao SP 6, Taixi KI 3 or tender areas close to them.

*Dizziness and dazzling visual disturbance*

Principal sites: head, Ganshu BL 18, Shenshu BL 23.

Add Taiyang, Shangyintang (1 cun below Yintang). Points on the Gall Bladder channel and on the temporo-parietal area.

*Dysmenorrhoea*

Principal sites: both sides of the lumbar and sacral spine, and the Ren Mai and KI channel pathways.

Main points: Qihai Ren 6 and Guanyuan Ren 4.
Additional points: Ganshu BL 18 and Sanyinjiao SP 6.

*Infantile convulsions*

Principal sites: Shixuan. The 12 Jing points of the hands may also be used, or Fengchi GB 20, Dazhui Du 14 and Shenzhu Du 12.

*Eye diseases*

Principal sites: points around the eye.

Ganshu BL 18, Danshu BL 19, Shenshu BL 23.

Add Fengchi GB 20 and Zanzhu BL 2 for glaucoma.

Add Fengchi GB 20, Tongziliao GB 1 for cataract.

Add Taiyang or Tongziliao GB 1, Zanzhu BL 2 for conjunctivitis.

*Blocked nose, sinusitis*

Principal sites: Feishu BL 13, Fengchi GB 20, Yingxiang LI 20.

When the nose has just become blocked Yingxiang LI 20 and Shangyingxiang (extra), 5 fen below LI 20, may be needled.

For sinusitis add Hegu LI 4 and Yuji LU 10.

*Tuberculosis in the lymph nodes* (Luoli)

Principal sites: both sides of the spine from T5–T10.

Needle around the tuberculous node.

## Contraindications

Acute infectious diseases, burns, cutaneous ulcers, acute abdominal disorders.

## Duration and frequency of treatment

The patient should be treated once a day or every other day. The course should last for 10–15 sessions and may be repeated once.

## RETAINED INTRADERMAL NEEDLE (Pi Nei Zhen)

Intradermal needles (Pi Nei Zhen) or 'embedding needles' (Mai Zhen) derive from an ancient technique where the needles were left in place. The technique consists of securing a small needle at a point in the skin, and leaving it there for an extended period.

This technique is used in diseases which require superficial stimulation and needle retention of long duration. It is also used in auriculotherapy.

### Equipment

Several types of needle may be used:

1. 'Grain of wheat' needle: 32 or 34 gauge tip, 1.5 cm long, and a very small handle, half the size of a grain of rice (Fig. 7.4),
2. Intradermal tack: same gauge, but shaped like a drawing pin (Fig. 7.4),
3. Standard acupuncture needle, 32 or 34 gauge and 5 fen long.

### Method

The needles should be sterilised, and the skin disinfected thoroughly.

#### 'Grain of wheat' needle

*Insertion.* Hold the body of the needle with a pair of tweezers in your right hand, stretching the skin around the point with your left hand. Position the needle so it is perpendicular to the flow of the channel, and at an angle of 15° to the skin, and insert. The needle should end up horizontal, 0.5–1 cm under the skin.

Example: Feishu BL 13 is on the back, on the inner Bladder line of Tai Yang. The channel flows downwards, so the needle should be inserted across it from right to left or from left to right, to make a right angle with the channel.

*Securing the needle.* When the needle has been inserted, place a small square of sticking plaster (1 cm × 1 cm) underneath the handle and the part of the body of the needle protruding from the skin. Next cover the needle with another, slightly larger, square of plaster. One of the corners of the plaster should be placed directly over the upper end of the handle.

Securing the needle in this way firstly prevents it from slipping when the patient moves, and secondly facilitates withdrawing the needle. All you need to do is lift the corner of the plaster opposite the handle and pull both away at the same time (Fig. 7.5).

#### Intradermal tack

The intradermal tack is used primarily on the face, the ears and those places where a superficial perpendicular insertion is required.

Hold the needle by its circular head, and secure the point to be needled. Hold the needle over the point and insert it by pushing down on its head, giving it a slight twist. Secure the needle with a small piece of sticking plaster. Another method is

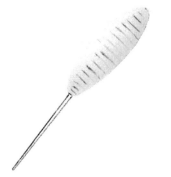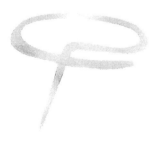

Fig. 7.4   Retained intradermal needles: 'grain of wheat' needle and intradermal tack.

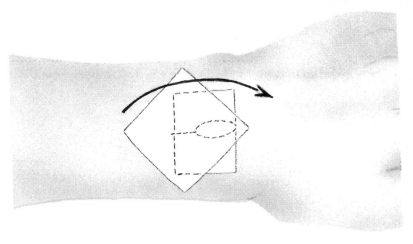

**Fig. 7.5**  Securing the 'grain of wheat' needle.

to use the tweezers to put the needle onto a small piece of sticking plaster. Hold the plaster by its edges and insert the needle, pushing on its head.

### Standard acupuncture needle

Insert the needle a few fen horizontally into the skin. The direction of insertion and method of securing the needle are the same as for the 'grain of wheat' needle.

### Duration of insertion

Retain intradermal needles as long as is required by the condition of the disease; this is generally a day or two, but it can be extended to a week. In summertime or in a hot environment this period should not exceed 48 hours. In winter the needles can be retained for 5–7 days.

### Indications

Intradermal needles are used to treat pain, such as headache, migraine, gastric pain and biliary colic, or chronic problems, such as insomnia, asthma, arterial hypertension, neurasthenia, menstrual disorders, urinary incontinence, Bi syndrome (Bi Zheng).

### Contraindications and precautions

— Before using an intradermal needle, check it carefully to make sure it will not fracture under the skin.

— Do not insert intradermal needles into points where they will inhibit the patient's movements. They should not be used in cases of inflammation, cutaneous ulcer or swelling.

— Withdraw the needle if the pain gets worse after insertion.

— Withdraw the needle if localised redness, swelling, weeping of fluids or signs of infection appear after insertion.

## TRIANGULAR NEEDLE (San Leng Zhen)

The triangular needle was developed from the fourth type of ancient needle (Feng — pointed, with a cutting edge), described in the *Ling Shu*, Chapter 1 (see above, Ch. 1).

Triangular needle technique consists of making a superficial tear in an area of skin or piercing a small vein to draw a small amount of blood. Bleeding has been common in China for a very long time and was performed with a needle made of stone (Bian Shi). The principles of its use were described in the ancient texts.

*Su Wen* (Ch. 24): 'When the particular energy affecting a vessel has been diagnosed, the physician should start with bleeding, which will expel the energy'.

*Ling Shu* (Ch. 1): 'Bleeding drains accumulation'.

*Ling Shu* (Ch. 7): 'Needling the collaterals with Luo technique dissipates blockages of blood'.

*Ling Shu* (Ch. 39): 'If there is congestion in the Luo, the congested area can be as small as the head of a pin or as big and long as a rope. In these cases the physician should draw some blood immediately'.

*Ling Shu* (Ch. 78): 'Bleeding disperses Heat'.

The triangular needle has a mode of action corresponding to 'bleeding the channels' (Ci Xue Luo) and 'draining Heat' (Chu Xue Xie Re). Bleeding 'opens the orifices and disperses Heat' (Kai Qiao Xie Re), and 'activates the Blood and disperses swellings' (Huo Xue Xiao Zhong). The triangular needle is therefore indicated in all cases of blockage in the channels, and in diseases with stagnation of Blood blocking the circulation.

*Bleeding with a triangular needle activates the Blood, dissolves stagnation of Blood, reduces inflammation, eases pain, disperses Fullness and eliminates Accumulation.*

## Equipment

The triangular needle is large, 2–3 cun long. The body has a triangular tip with 3 extremely sharp edges. A hypodermic needle, razor blade or cutaneous needle (Pi Fu Zhen) can be used instead.

## Method

There are 5 different ways of using the triangular needle. Before proceeding, carefully disinfect your hands and the area to be treated. Sterilise the needle.

### Swift needling (Dian Ci)

Hold the area to be needled firmly with your left hand in tiger claw. Hold the needle between the thumb, index and third fingers of your right hand and aim it precisely towards the vessel or point. Insert the needle rapidly $\frac{1}{2}$ or 1 fen deep, then withdraw it straight away. The point should bleed, and should not be staunched. If no blood comes out, press gently around the hole to help the stagnant blood move. Finish off the operation by pressing on the hole with a sterile gauze to stop the bleeding. When needling a superficial vein, press along the vein to induce local congestion of blood around the area to be needled.

*Indications:*

— Lumbar pain caused by accumulation of blood following external trauma: needle Weizhong BL 54.

— Pain and swelling of the throat: needle Shaoshang LU 11.

— Diarrhoea and vomiting in acute gastroenteritis: needle Quchi LI 11, Weizhong BL 54.

— Acute conjunctivitis: needle Taiyang (extra) or Erjian LI 2.

— Sunstroke (Zhong Shu) and stroke (closed Zhong Feng): needle the 10 Xuan.

— In cases of children suffering from Ganji (diseases arising from malnutrition with emaciation, dyspepsia, diarrhoea, swelling of the abdomen with thin limbs): needle the Sifeng (extra) points.

— Redness and swelling of the joints in Hot Bi (Re Bi): needle local points.

### Dispersed needling (San Ci)

This is also known as 'leopardskin needling' (Bao Wen Ci).

Mark out the affected area by bleeding in different locations around it: in front, behind, to the right and to the left of the inflammation, or along the edges of the redness.

*Indications.* This technique is used in skin diseases and in conditions which cover a large area, for example:

— sprain,
— rebellious dermatosis,
— cutaneous ulcers. In these cases needle directly into the ulcer or use San Ci technique around it.

Generally the patient is needled 2–8 times. A cutaneous needle (Pi Fu Zhen) may be used, but only with moderate bleeding.

### Tearing (Tiao Ci)

This technique consists of inducing some bleeding by tearing a little piece of skin with the tip of the triangular needle.

Pinch the skin with your left hand. With your right hand insert the needle rapidly to a depth of $\frac{1}{2}$ fen, then immediately lean the needle over. As the point lifts up it will tear the skin. Allow a little blood to flow. If there is no blood, squeeze the area around the tear with the thumb and index fingers of both hands. The blood should come out straight away.

*Indications:*

— Multiple sycosis, especially with boils on the nape of the neck: look for red points on either side of the spine and bleed with a triangular needle.

— Haemorrhoids: bleed any brown points on the lumbo-sacral area.

— Gan Ji (infantile malnutrition): bleed the Sifeng extra points.

### Cluster needling (Cong Ci)

Use swift needling (Dian Ci), keeping the locations grouped closely together and over a limited area, and leave to bleed.

*Indications.* This type of bleeding is usually used in combination with cupping for the following:

— sprains
— Bi syndrome
— alopecia
— ulcers.

### Circular needling (Wei Ci)

Needle swiftly around a painful or swollen area.

## Points commonly treated with triangular needles

### Shixuan (10 extra points on the fingertips)

Technique: Dian Ci, bleed.
    Indications: hyperpyrexia, fainting, sunstroke, syncope, paresis of the hands and feet.

### Shi'er Jing (12 Jing points on the fingertips)

Technique: Dian Ci, bleed.
    Indications: hyperpyrexia, fainting, sore throat, tonsillitis.

### Sifeng (extra points)

Technique: Dian Ci, needle the points and squeeze until a little yellowish fluid comes out.

Indications: poor digestion, indigestion, whooping cough, Gan Ji (infantile malnutrition).

### Yuji LU 10

Technique: Dian Ci or San Ci, bleed.
    Indications: hyperpyrexia, sore throat, tonsillitis.

### Chize LU 5

Technique: Dian Ci, bleed.
    Indications: sunstroke, vomiting and acute diarrhoea.

### Quze P 3

Technique: Dian Ci, bleed.
    Indications: sunstroke, oppression of the chest, uneasy feeling with sensations of oppression, heat in the chest and suffocation (Xin Fan: usually translated as 'anxious agitation').

### Weizhong BL 54

Technique: Dian Ci, bleed.
    Indications: sunstroke, vomiting and acute diarrhoea, contracture of the calf.

### Bafeng (extra points)

Technique: Dian Ci, bleed.
    Indications: paresis, painful swelling of the feet.

### Baxie (extra points)

Technique: Dian Ci, bleed.
    Indications: painful swelling and paresis of the hand.

### Yintang (extra)

Technique: Dian Ci, bleed.
    Indications: headache, dizziness, fainting, red eyes and rhinitis.

### Taiyang (extra)

Technique: Dian Ci or San Ci, bleed.
    Indications: headache, red and sore eyes.

*Baihui Du 20*

Technique: Dian Ci, bleed.

Indications: headache, fainting, dizziness, dazzling visual disturbance, arterial hypertension.

*Erjian, Pingjian, Erbei* (extra points)

Technique: Dian Ci, bleed.

Indications: hyperpyrexia, tonsillitis, red and sore eyes, arterial hypertension.

*Jinjin, Yuye* (extra points)

Technique: Dian Ci, bleed.

Indications: stroke (Zhong Feng), stiff tongue, speech difficulties.

## Contraindications

Do not use triangular needles in Blood Deficiency (Empty blood) syndromes (Xue Xu Zheng), in cases of hypotension, on patients with a weak constitution, pregnant women, women after childbirth, patients on anti-coagulant therapy or people suffering from spontaneous or chronic bleeding.

## Precautions

1. Explain the technique to the patient so that he does not faint when he sees blood.

2. Perform the technique gently and superficially. Avoid causing too much bleeding.

3. Carefully disinfect your hands as well as the area to be treated. Sterilise the needle. If the bleeding is excessive, press down on the point with a gauze to stop the bleeding.

4. Needle once a day, or once every other day. If a lot of blood is lost do not needle more than twice a week.

## LONG NEEDLE (Mang Zhen)

The long needle is a filiform needle, long 'like a beard of wheat', used in chronic diseases where deep needling is required. This needle originates from the eighth type of ancient needle (Chang), described in Chapter 1 of the *Ling Shu* (see above, Ch. 1).

## Equipment

A 29–32 gauge filiform needle with a body length of 5 cun, 7 cun, 1 chi, 1 chi 5 cun, 2 chi, 2 chi 5 cun, or 3 chi (16–96 cm).

## Method

*Insertion.* Fold over the third, fourth and fifth fingers of your left hand and press firmly on the skin to stop it from moving. Hold the body of the needle with the thumb and index finger of your left hand and insert it, turning it gently at the same time. Simultaneously rotate the handle of the needle with the thumb, index and third fingers of your right hand. As the needle penetrates, both hands should work in concert, steadily rotating the needle (Fig. 7.6 and see above, Ch. 2, Fig. 2.14).

*Reinforcing and Reducing.* There are no particular techniques of reinforcing or reducing. The needle is withdrawn as soon as Qi is obtained.

When needling the limbs, the back, the head and the face, the angle of rotation should be large in Full syndromes, and small in Empty syndromes.

*Depth and direction of insertion.* Depth of insertion is determined by the precise moment when the patient feels needle sensation.

Points on the abdomen and the sides of the abdomen can be needled straight. For points on the midline of the abdomen, needle to a depth of 7 or 8 cun. If the sensation arrives at a depth of 4 or 5 cun, however, there is no need to continue advancing the needle. On the Dai Mai channel, situated on the border of the abdomen, needle to a depth of roughly 1 chi 2 cun–2 chi. Below the waist on the buttocks, needle obliquely to a depth of 5–8 cun. On the back, the thorax and areas over vital organs close to the surface such as the heart, lungs, liver and spleen, needle horizontally and superficially. On the head and face 'needle swiftly' (Dianci).

## Indications

The long needle is indicated mainly in chronic diseases: rheumatic pain, menstrual disorders, mental diseases, intestinal diseases, or in diseases which have not improved in response to short needles.

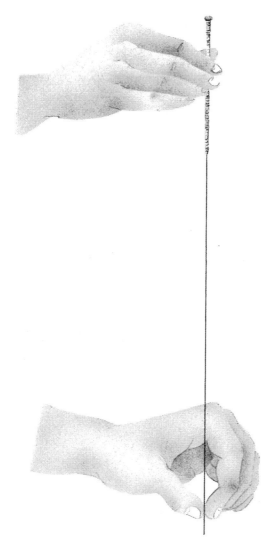

**Fig. 7.6** The long needle.

## Contraindications

- Body weakened by chronic disease,
- Hypersensitivity,
- Swollen areas,
- Progressive skin disease,
- Pregnancy,
- Children and adolescents.

## Observations

1. Using the long needle requires a great deal of experience. Always treat your patients with other techniques first, turning to the long needle only as a last resort.

2. The length of the needle will frighten some patients, and it is important to explain the kind of sensation they will experience. The needle should be inserted gradually so that the reaction is slow. Do not manipulate it abruptly or the patient may faint.

3. The patient must lie flat in a comfortable position so he does not move during treatment.

4. To avoid injury, do not needle too deep on the trunk, particularly over the internal organs.

## WARM NEEDLE (Wen Zhen)

This technique combines the effects of needling with moxibustion, and uses either mugwort or hot wax.

When moxa is burned on the needle, the heat follows the pathway of the channel more closely than in other kinds of moxibustion; with direct or indirect moxa cones and moxa sticks, the heat spreads more diffusely.

### Warm needle with mugwort

Insert the needle, obtain Qi, reinforce or reduce according to the requirements of the treatment, then leave the needle in place. Prepare a ball of moxa, separate it into two halves and join them over the handle of the needle.

A 1 or 2 cm slice from a moxa stick may be used instead of the ball of moxa, and should be pushed onto the handle. Leave at least 2 cm between the skin and the base of the moxa or piece of moxa stick.

Take a 5 × 5 cm piece of paper and tear it diagonally halfway across. Do not cut with scissors. Hold the two sides of the tear apart and slide the paper on either side of the needle to cover the point. Use an incense stick to light the ball or slice of moxa at the base, so that the heat is conducted straight down through the needle (Fig. 7.7).

### Precautions

Use a 26 gauge needle. The moxa should be the size of a broad bean. Be sure to compress the moxa punk well with your fingers, smoothing down the outer surface so nothing falls off.

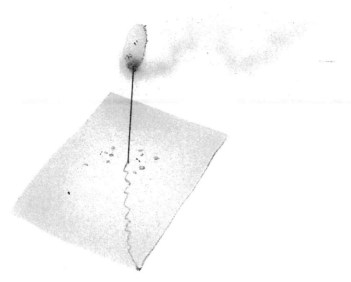

**Fig. 7.7** Warm needle with mugwort.

The paper has a dual purpose: it collects the ash, and protects the skin from the heat radiating from the moxa.

On no account should the patient move. Do not use warm needle in cases where the needle is not to be retained.

### Warm needle with wax

This technique consists of retaining the needle and warming it with molten wax.

Prepare a needle and a small ampoule (the type used for storing antibiotics) filled with paraffin wax. Heat this in a 'bain marie' (double boiler) till the wax is liquid.

Leave the wax to cool for about 10 minutes, until the sides of the ampoule begin to look like frosted glass. The centre of the wax will still be liquid and at the right temperature, between 48° and 52°C. The temperature of the wax is quite stable, and will only drop about 2° during the treatment. It cannot damage the skin or tissues.

Whilst the wax is cooling select a point and insert the needle. When Qi sensation has been obtained reinforce or reduce as required then leave the needle in place.

Insert the handle and part of the body of the needle into the ampoule, so that the opening is about 1 cm from the skin. Hold the ampoule still or rotate it.

The patient will rapidly experience continuous sensations of stinging, numbness, distension, heaviness, heat and diffusion. The most pronounced sensations will generally be distension, heaviness and heat. Remove the ampoule after 10 minutes, reheat and prepare to use again. 30 minutes of continuous application will maintain the needle sensation. Remove the needle.

It is imperative to obtain Qi sensation before applying any warm needle techniques. If Qi has not appeared at the needle, warming it will not achieve the desired effect.

### Indications

Flaccid paralysis, Wind, Cold and Damp Bi, Cold stagnation in the channels and collaterals, Qi and Blood stagnation, paresis, numbness, diarrhoea, abdominal distension, Emptiness and Cold in the Stomach and Spleen.

### FIRE NEEDLE (Huo Zhen)

This technique involves heating a large needle until it is red hot, then inserting it swiftly into the point.

The needle used for this technique has been developed from the Da (big) needle described in the *Ling Shu*, Chapter 1 (see above, Ch.1).

This technique is called 'quenching' in the *Nei Jing* (Cui Ci), after the practice of quenching iron in a forge. There are many references to the use of fire needles in the classics, for example:

*Ling Shu* (Ch. 7): 'Fire needle treats Bi syndrome'.

*Qian Jin Yi Fang*: 'Fire needle is used to treat boil, carbuncle, and skin ulcers'.

This technique 'warms the channels, disperses cold' (Wen Jing San Han), and 'clears the channels, invigorates the collaterals' (Tong Jing Huo Luo).

## Equipment

The needles used today are 26 or 27 gauge and made of stainless steel. They should be firm and flexible. Copper needles are good heat conductors, but tend to get soft after a while: they are therefore not recommended. The body of the fire needle is quite large, ranging from 0.5 mm (26 or 27 gauge) to 1 mm in diameter. They are 1–2 cun long. If the needle is too long it is difficult to use, as it bends easily. If the needle is short the handle must be insulated with a piece of bamboo or a pad of cotton wool. This is not necessary for longer needles.

## Method

Disinfect the area to be needled. If the patient is very sensitive inject the area with a local anaesthetic of 2–10% procaine solution. 0.2% adrenalin chlorhydrate may be added to prevent haemorrhaging.

### Deep needling (Shen Ci)

Hold the needle in your right hand, securing the area to be treated with your left hand in tiger claw. Sometimes the left thumbnail may be pressed into the edge of the point. Heat the needle progressively until it is red hot, working from the handle towards the tip, and insert it swiftly, withdrawing it immediately. Massage the point with a pad of cotton wool. Depth of insertion should be approximately 5 fen–1 cun.

### Superficial needling (Qian Ci)

When the needle is red hot, insert it skin-deep only.

A cutaneous needle (Pi Fu Zhen) can be used. Heat the spines until they are red hot then tap the area to be treated.

## Choice of points

The principles are the same as for the filiform needle (Hao Zhen), and the choice of points is made according to the symptoms of the disease, the constitution and the age of the patient.

Usually only a few points are needled, though more may be used in Full syndromes (Excess) and on young and robust patients. The points selected should generally be on or close to the diseased area, or Ashi points.

Depth of insertion is determined by the thickness of the musculature and the location of blood vessels at the point. Usually needling is deeper on the limbs, the abdomen and the lumbar region (2–5 fen), and more superficial on the chest and back (1–2 fen).

## Indications

The fire needle is used for cases of tuberculous lymph node, carbuncle, urticaria, warts, flat condyloma, naevi, and in Cold Bi Syndrome (Han Bi), gastric pain and prolapse, diarrhoea, impotence, irregular menstruation, dysmenorrhoea, Gan Ji (infantile malnutrition), mastitis.

If the practitioner is trying to discharge pus a large diameter needle should be used. Conversely, a finer needle is recommended to break up Yin type swellings and hard masses.

## Precautions

Heat the needle progressively, starting with the body and finishing with the tip. Do not insert the needle if the body is hot but the tip has cooled. This conforms to the recommendations in the Fire Needle chapter in the *Zhen Jiu Da Cheng*: 'To be effective the needle is heated until it is red hot. If it is not red hot the disease will not be expelled; indeed, the patient will be harmed'.

The points should be precisely located. The practitioner should avoid blood vessels, tendons and bones. The movement is swift and precise, and the needle should be withdrawn as soon as the diseased area has been reached. Remember the recommendations of the *Zhen Jiu Da Cheng* (Fire Needle chapter): 'Under no circumstances should needling be too deep so that no injury is caused to the vessels, but if the needling is too superficial it will not expel the disease'.

The fire needle should be used with caution on the face, as it may leave small scars. The *Zhen Jiu Da Cheng* (Fire Needle chapter) says: 'The physician can use a fire needle anywhere on the body, but he should be very careful and avoid using it on the face'.

Do not use fire needle in cases of hyperpyrexia.

If redness, swelling or itching appear at the point within a few days of treatment, particular attention should be paid to asepsis during treatment.

## PAEDIATRIC NEEDLES (Er Zhen)

There are several types of needle which can be used on children: a 34 gauge 0.5 cun filiform needle, a cutaneous needle (Pi Fu Zhen) or its substitute, the 'hard toothbrush', which have already been studied in this chapter.

There is, however, a type of needle used exclusively in paediatrics, which despite its considerable importance is unfamiliar to many acupuncturists. The following directions explain how to make one and how to use it (Fig. 7.8).

### Materials

— A glass pipette tube with an external dia-meter of 5 mm and an internal diameter of 2.3–2.5 mm. Length when complete: 5 cm, but several spare lengths may be necessary for unsuccessful attempts.

— For the actual needle: a cylinder of 14 carat white gold, 2.8 cm long, 2.2 mm in diameter. The tip of the needle should be professionally sharpened into a candle shape about 5 mm long. The tapered tip of the 'candle' should measure 2 mm, and be chamfered so there are no sharp edges. These instructions follow the standards for grinding for commercial disposable needles.

— 2 10 carat gold cylinders for counterweights, 5 mm long, 2.2 mm in diameter.

### Construction

Half close one end of the glass tube with a Bunsen burner.

Slide the counterweights through the other end into the tube, then insert the needle, base first.

Partly close the end of the tube from which the tip of the needle protrudes with the Bunsen burner. The edges of the tube, tightened by the heat into a small circular opening, should fit the curve of the 'candle' perfectly. If the tube is held vertically, tip pointing downwards, the tip should protrude about 2 mm.

Several attempts may be needed to obtain the desired result. Discard anything which is less than perfect.

**NB:** To cut the pipette tube into sections, file it

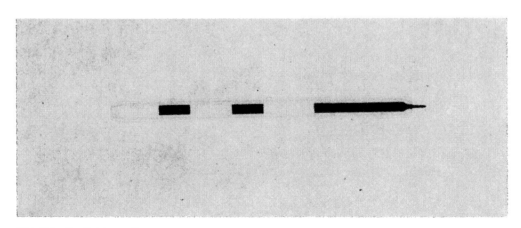

**Fig. 7.8** Paediatric needle.

to the desired length with a glasscutter (triangular file) and snap it with your hands.

## Practice and use

To practise, place the cushion in front of you angled at 45° to the right.

Hold the needle by the blunt end with your thumb and index finger, exactly between the pads of each finger. The end of the tube should not protrude upwards beyond the fingers but is buried between the fingertips.

Starting from the distal end of the cushion and working towards you, tap from one end to the other with your hand. The tapping should be light and springy, with a dozen impacts in under 3 seconds.

During this movement the end of the tube strikes the surface to be treated lightly and the tip of the needle acts on the surface of the skin, causing no pain whatsoever for the patient.

Practice should continue until the percussive movement of the hand is automatic and the strokes flow together evenly without being dragged down by the weight of the hand.

This technique is recommended for the treatment of children under the age of seven.

Treat the entire length of Ren Mai, the inner Bladder line, the internal and external aspects of the forearm, and the internal and external aspects of the leg. You may finish with three strokes on selected points, especially Neiguan P 6, Sanyinjiao SP 6, Waiguan TB 5, Zusanli ST 36.

# 8. Cupping (Ba Guan Zi)

A cupping jar or cup is a small bottle with a smooth and rounded mouth used to create a partial vacuum over the skin. This causes the blood to circulate and pulls it towards the surface of the body.

'Jiao Fa' is the ancient term used to describe cupping jars, indicating that the early types were made of animal horns. With the passage of time, they have been made of all sorts of materials, and numerous techniques have been devised to evacuate the air from the cup.

## Types

Cups come in a wide variety of sizes and materials. The ones most commonly used are made of glass, earthenware or bamboo. Copper or iron cups are also used. Glass cups being transparent, the practitioner can see the degree of congestion on the skin and adjust the length of treatment accordingly. On the other hand they conduct heat too easily and are fragile. Most importantly, the rim of the cup should be very smooth. The diameter of the mouth is usually 1 cun, 1 cun 5 fen, or 2 cun. Earthenware cups have long necks and large volumes, so their suction is very strong.

## Methods

### Preparation

There are several different methods for removing the air from the cup.

### 1. Combustion

**a. Tou Huo Fa**. Fold a small square of paper into a cone (Fig. 8.1a). Light one end and drop the burning cone into the cup (Fig. 8.1b). The burning paper will expel the air, creating a partial vacuum. Place the cup upside down onto the area to be treated (Fig. 8.1c).

**b. Tie Mian Fa**. Moisten a small pad of cotton wool with alcohol, squeeze it flat into a pill shape and press it onto the inner surface of the cup. Light, allow to burn for a moment, then place the cup over the area to be treated.

**c. Shan Huo Fa**. Moisten a scrap of cotton wool with alcohol and light. Hold the cup in your left hand. With your right hand use some tweezers to move the cotton wool around inside the cup then put it in position (Fig. 8.2). If it does not stay in place put the burning swab back inside the cup and position it a second time. Cotton buds on cardboard sticks are very convenient and may be used instead.

**d. Jia Huo Fa**. Use something non-flammable and heat conducting, for example a coin resting on a small disc of cardboard. Put this on the area to be treated, and place on it a small piece of cotton wool soaked in alcohol. Light it, and position the cup over it straight away, taking care not to overturn the base and burn the patient.

### 2. Boiling

Place the cups in boiling water for 10 minutes, then take them out with tweezers and shake them to empty out all the water. Next tap the rim gently against a piece of towelling soaked in cold water and quickly place the cup down flat over the point or area to be treated.

### Removal

The optimum duration of treatment is between 3

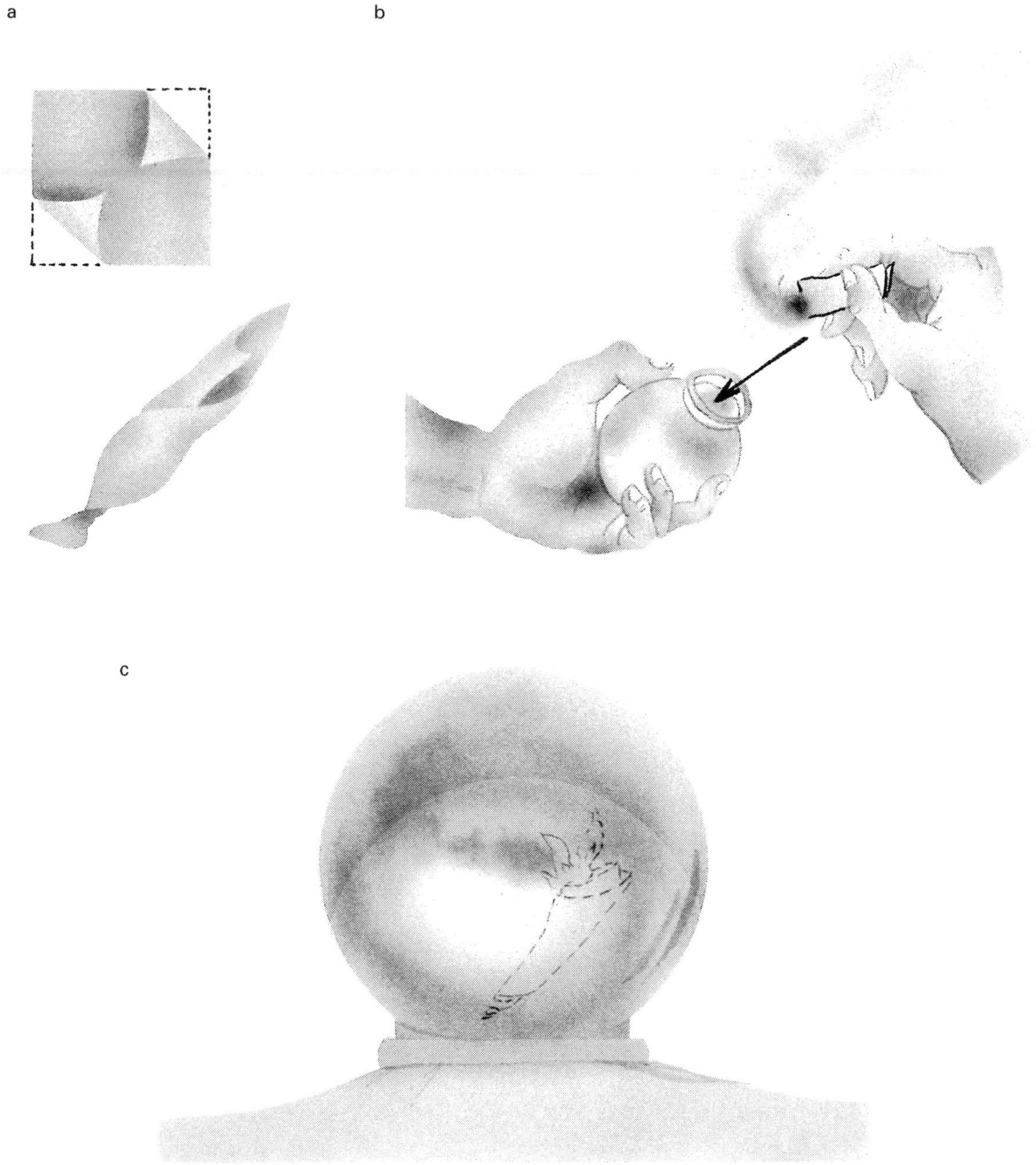

a

b

c

**Fig. 8.1a–c** Preparation: Tou Huo technique. **a** Fold paper. **b** Light paper. **c** Put cup in position.

and 10 minutes, and should be adjusted according to the strength of the vacuum inside the cup.

When the process is complete remove the cup. Hold it in one hand and depress the skin around the mouth with the other hand to let in some air (Fig. 8.3).

## Applications

### 1. Simple cups and suction cups

*a. Simple cups*. Different types of cup can be used. The size varies according to the area to be treated and the nature of the disease.

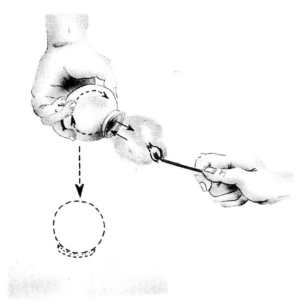

**Fig. 8.2** Preparation: Shan Huo technique.

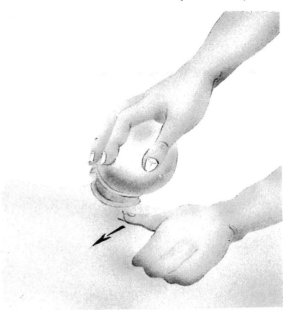

**Fig. 8.3** Removing the cup.

**b. Suction cups.** These are simple cups from which the air is pumped out, forming varying degrees of vacuum.

*Method*: Take an empty ampoule (the type used for storing intravenous antibiotics), cut off the base and rub the rim with sandpaper or a grindstone until completely smooth.

Select a point appropriate to the disease.

Place the ampoule over the point and press it against the skin. Use a 10 or 20 ml syringe to withdraw the air through the rubber stopper until the ampoule sticks tightly (Fig. 8.4). Inject 4–5 ml of water into the cup to lessen the vacuum and prevent bleeding.

Remove the cup after 10 or 15 minutes and wipe the point.

Seven sessions constitute a course of treatment, varying the points each time. The course may be extended for chronic diseases.

*Observations:*

— Do not use very strong suction when treating people with a weak constitution. Usually no more than 20 ml of air should be withdrawn.

— This technique is often used to ease the pain caused by acupuncture.

— When cupping older patients suffering from arterial hypertension, also needle Quchi LI 11 and Neiguan P 6.

**c. Indications for simple cups and suction cups:**

— Pain from Full Damp Heat, articular pain with accumulation of fluid on the joint
— Pains in the back and lumbar region (especially arising from Damp):

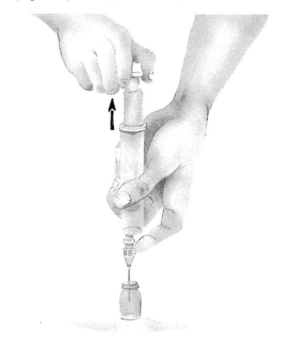

**Fig. 8.4** Suction cup.

Yinmen BL 51, Yaoyan (extra), Yaoyangguan Du 3, Dazhui Du 14
— Headache:
Dazhui Du 14, Taiyang (extra), Yintang (extra)
— Chronic gastric pain:
Zhongwan Ren 12, Weishu BL 21, Zusanli ST 36
— Abdominal pain from attack of Cold or indigestion:
Sanyinjiao SP 6, Guanyuan Ren 4
— Abdominal pain in children:
Shenque Ren 8
— Diarrhoea:
Tianshu ST 25, Qihai Ren 6, Zusanli ST 36
— Ganmao (colds, flu, upper respiratory tract infection):
Dazhui Du 14, Dashu BL 11, Hegu LI 4
— Cough:
Feishu BL 13, Dingshuan (extra), Geshu BL 17
— Asthma:
Zhongfu LU 1, Qihai Ren 6, Fengmen BL 12
— Painful chest and sides:
Zhangmen LIV 13, Yanglinquan GB 34, Tianyingxue (extra)
— Dysmenorrhoea:
Daimai GB 26, Yinjiao Ren 7, Xuehai SP 10
— Arterial hypertension:
Jianyu LI 15, Quchi LI 11, Hegu LI 4, Chengfu BL 50, Weizhong BL 54, Chengjin BL 56, Kunlun BL 60, Yongquan KI 1, Shenmai BL 62, Zusanli ST 36.

**d. Precautions.** Cups are retained for varying lengths of time. They should be removed when the skin has gone purple, which usually takes about 5 minutes. If the skin has not gone red after 5 minutes, the treatment is not appropriate. The quicker the skin goes red, the better the prognosis.

Do not use too many cups at a time.

### 2. Migration cupping (Tui Guan Fa)

Withdraw the air from the cup using Shan Huo Fa technique until it sticks to the area to be treated.

Apply a thin layer of lubricant around the cup and on the edge of the mouth (vaseline, vegetable oil, or water in summertime). Rotate the cup clockwise (Fig. 8.5a), moving it all over the affected area (Fig. 8.5b), until this goes reddish purple. Use both hands to move the cup, lifting the base slightly in the direction required (Fig. 8.5c, d).

This technique is used on areas which are quite extensive, and where the musculature is quite thick. It is therefore very good for back and spinal pain.

### 3. Cups with medication (Yao Guan Fa)

There are several techniques:

**a. Impregnated cups.** Prepare a decoction of the following formula (wrap all the ingredients in some muslin). Take 6 g each of:

*Herba Ephedra*
*Angelica pubescens*
*Ledebourellia divaricata*
*Chaenomeles lagenaria*
*Zantoxyllum piperitum*
*Gentiana macrophylla*
*Datura metel*
*Artemisia anomala*
*Boswellia carterii*
*Commiphora myrrha*
*Notopterygium incisum.*

Place some bamboo cups in the decoction and boil for 15 minutes. The cups should now be applied using 'boiling' technique. The main indications for impregnated cups are pain arising from Wind Damp (Feng Shi Tong).

**b. Cups with medicated solution.** A medicinal solution is placed inside a simple or suction cup, for example:

- Pepper water (*Capsicum frutescens*)
- Tincture of *Zanthoxylum nitidum*
- Fresh ginger juice
- Feng Shi alcohol (*Syzygum aromaticum, Ilex chinensis, Eucalyptus globulus, Cinnamomum camphora . . .*).

Medicine cups are indicated in pains arising from Wind Damp, cough, asthma, colds, chronic gastritis, digestive problems and psoriasis.

### 4. Cupping over a needle (Zhen Guan Fa)

When the acupuncture needle has been inserted

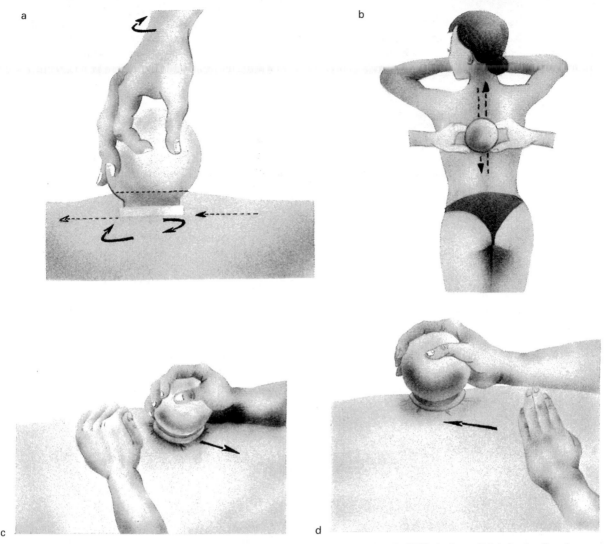

**Fig. 8.5a–d** Moving the cup. **a** Rotating the cup. **b** Moving the cup on the back. **c & d** Lift the base slightly in the direction required.

and Qi has been obtained, place the cup over the needle. This technique is often used for pains arising from Wind Damp.

*5. Scarification cupping*

**a. Bleeding with a triangular needle.** Needle the affected area swiftly (Dian Ci) with a triangular needle and make it bleed. To increase the bleeding expel the air from a cup and put it on the point.

**b. Bleeding with a scalpel**

*Equipment*: scalpel, various sized cups, cotton wool soaked in alcohol.

*Choice of points*: the points may be close to the affected area, or Ashi points.

*Stage 1*: Bleeding with the scalpel.

Disinfect the area to be treated.

Hold the scalpel vertically with your right hand, third finger on the tip. Needle the skin swiftly (Dian Ci) several times in a straight line, without drawing the scalpel across the skin. The length of the incision should be shorter than the diameter of the mouth of the cup, and no deeper than is necessary to draw some blood. There should be a gap the width of a grain of rice between each incision.

30–40 incisions are made for large-sized cups, 20–25 for medium sizes, and 10–15 for small ones. The depth of the incision is determined by the nature of the diseased area and the thickness of the musculature. Blood vessels must be avoided.

*Stage 2*: Applying the cup.

This is the most important part of the technique, and determines its success.

Use a piece of burning cotton wool or a piece of paper folded into a cone. Set light to the top third and put it into the cup. Take a deep breath, lean the cup over the affected area and blow into the mouth to fill it full of oxygen. Blow continuously until the paper is burning merrily with a blue flame. Quickly put the cup onto the skin.

*Stage 3*: Removing the cup.

Retain the cup for 5–10 minutes. Press on the skin by the edge of the cup and blow some air inside. Wipe the lines of blood with a sterile gauze and apply a dressing.

*Frequency of treatment.* Leave a gap of 3–10 days between sessions. A course of treatment usually comprises 4–6 sessions.

*Observations.* Use 2 or 3 cups for the first session, and 2–5 cups for subsequent sessions. Do not use more than 6 cups at a time. The number of cups is determined by the constitution of the patient and the condition of the disease.

Use this technique in conjunction with other methods to treat venomous snakebite, chilblain, sprain, or neurodermatitis.

## Contraindications

Hyperpyrexia, spasm, convulsion, ulceration of the skin, skin allergies, cardiac failure, malignant tumour, progressive pulmonary tuberculosis, mental disease, haemorrhagic disease, acute infectious disease. Cupping should not be applied during menstruation, on weak and old patients, or on the abdominal or the lumbar region of pregnant women.

## Observations

1. The patient should be comfortable so that he stays still during the treatment.

2. Do not cup emaciated parts of the body, bony areas, blood vessels, varicose veins, and previous sites of cupping which are still congestive and where the blood has not yet been resorbed.

3. Migration cupping should be performed slowly.

4. When cupping over a needle instruct the patient not to tense his muscles.

5. Scarification cupping should not draw more than 10 centilitres of blood.

# 9. Manual techniques

Manual techniques are a simple form of therapy used today by most people in China before they resort to an acupuncturist. They can be thought of as therapy for the family.

The most commonly used techniques are acupressure, pushing and rolling, and friction.

## ACUPRESSURE (Zhi Zhen Liao Fa)

Acupressure, or stimulation with the fingers, is a simple but effective therapeutic technique which consists of massaging acupuncture points with the fingers. It has been in popular use for a long time. The *Zhen Jiu Da Cheng* says 'Pinch the tendons on both arms (hands) if the person has a sudden seizure (Jijing), and collapses as if dead'.

Acupressure is suitable for the elderly, for women and children, for people who are frightened of needles, and in emergencies when there are no needles to hand.

### Techniques

Four different techniques are commonly used:

*1. Pressing* (Dian Qia)

Press the pad of your thumb perpendicularly down on the point. Either gentle or strong stimulation can be applied. To give gentle stimulation, press your thumb down a little, withdraw it straight away, then press again. To give strong stimulation, press your thumb in firmly and deeply, leave it at that level for a while, partially withdraw it, then press in deep again. In both cases use rhythmic pressure.

Gentle pressure is used in cases of weakness following chronic disease, on places where the musculature is thin and on children and the elderly. Strong pressure is used in cases of acute disease and loss of consciousness, on places where the musculature is thick and on people with a strong constitution.

*2. Pressing over an area* (Dian Kou)

Pressing with one finger gives strong stimulation. Press the Shu points and the nerves with the middle finger of your right hand.

Pressing with several fingers gives gentle stimulation. Press with 3–5 fingers of one or both hands. Keep your fingers in a line or bunch them together into a 'plum blossom' shape. Press muscle groups (Jiqun) or the skull.

*3. Pressing and Picking Up* (An Ban)

Press with one finger and pick up in the opposite direction with the others. This technique stimulates the deeper nerves and tendons (Jijian).

*4. Pinching* (Nie Na)

Pinch with 3 fingers: thumb, index and third fingers. This technique stimulates the deep tendons (Jijian), muscle groups (Jiqun), or two symmetrical points, for example Quchi LI 11 and Shaohai HT 3, Neiguan P 6 and Waiguan TB 5.

Do not press suddenly or allow your nails to dig in during any of these techniques or you may cause discomfort to the patient. Increase the pressure gradually and massage all around the point, stopping when it becomes painful.

As most points form part of a pair, two

symmetrical points can be pressed at the same time, usually for 2–3 minutes.

### Choice of points

#### 1. Points on the channels

— Points on the channel pathways, on the limbs and the trunk, according to the location of the disease.
— The 'Huatuo' points, one finger's breadth lateral to the spine, on both sides.
— Standard points on the head, face, neck, nape of the neck and the limbs.

#### 2. Points on the peripheral nerve trunks

— Tender points over nerve plexi such as the subclavicular depression and the axilla.
— Points where the nerves are more superficial, for example around the joints of the limbs.
— Points in tender areas, for example around the nails, the plantar aspect of the joints of the foot and the palmar aspect of the joints of the hand.

#### 3. Points on the area affected by the disease

— Tender areas, atrophied muscle groups, or around a fracture which has mended.

### Indications

Acupressure has a broad range of applications. It can be used in any disease where acupuncture is indicated. It is often used in cases of pain such as headache, toothache and abdominal pain. It is also used for neurological problems affecting the sense organs.

### Contraindications

1. Acute infectious disease or high fever
2. Immediately after meals, after strenuous physical activity or sport
3. Skin disease, urticaria, pimples, ulceration, or inflammation near the point.

### Observations

1. The practitioner should keep his nails rounded and cut down to his fingertips. If they are too long they may dig into the skin; if they are too short the technique will be difficult to perform. The practitioner's hands should be warm, as cold hands can affect the treatment. He should disinfect his hands before starting.

2. For good results the intensity of the pressure should be adjusted to suit the patient. It may need to be firm or gentle, but the pressure should be consistent, not too fast and not too slow. Regular practice is necessary to learn to modulate the force of the wrist and fingers.

3. Make the patient comfortable and explain the technique to him so he feels relaxed.

## PUSHING AND ROLLING (Nie Ji Liao Fa)

This technique consists of rolling the tissues on either side of the spine. It is a massage technique (Tui Na).

### Method

The patient sits down leaning forwards, his hands on his temples, his back muscles relaxed. The practitioner stands behind him. The technique starts at the level of the sacrum.

Supinate both hands so that your thumbs are on top. With your index finger and thumb take hold

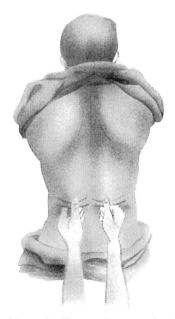

**Fig. 9.1** Pushing and rolling: supinate your hands so that your thumbs are on top.

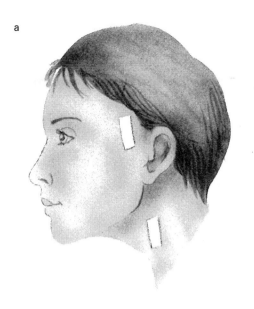

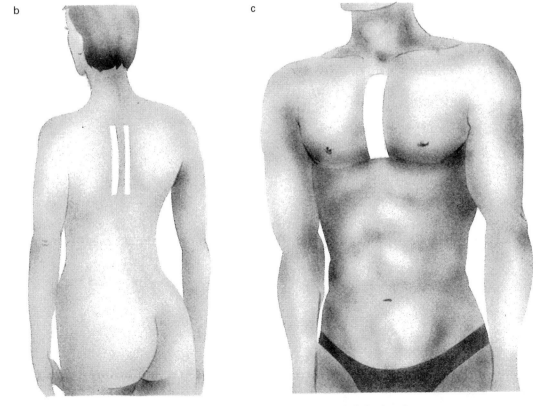

**Fig. 9.2a–c**   Friction: locations. **a** Head and neck. **b** Back. **c** Sternum.

of the skin and muscles on either side of the spine. Push upwards with your index fingers, and pinch, roll, pick up and pull the skin downwards with your thumbs (Fig. 9.1).

Both hands should work together, moving upwards from the sacrum as far as the cervix. Repeat the procedure 3–5 times, going upwards each time. On the second or third time pick the skin up at a slight diagonal. If the technique is practised correctly you should be able to hear a particular kind of sound on either side of L2 and L5. When you have finished, massage the following points gently 3 or 4 times with your thumbs: Feishu BL 13, Xinshu BL 15, Ganshu BL 18, Pishu BL 20 and Shenshu BL 23.

*Frequency of treatment.* Treat once daily for 6 days. If the disease is more serious start the treatment again for 12 days.

## Indications

This technique benefits the circulation in the channels, invigorates the Blood, and balances the digestive tract. In children it treats malnutrition, indigestion, stagnation of food or milk, and chronic gastroenteritis.

## FRICTION (Gua Sha Liao Fa)

Friction (Gua Sha) is a safe and effective form of therapy. In China it is commonly used by the general population, especially in the country, and is valued for its simplicity and freedom from side-effects. It is used to treat diseases of external origin (*Waigan*), headache, gastric and abdominal pain, asthma (*Chuanxiao*), sunstroke (*Zhongshu*) and oppression in the chest.

## Method

### Locations

- The Tai Yang area on the temple
- 2 locations about 2 cun lateral to and on either side of the Adam's apple (Fig. 9.2a)
- The inner Bladder line, between the spine and the inner border of the scapula, from the point level with the top of the scapula to the point level with the bottom (Fig. 9.2b)
- The midline of the chest, over the sternum (Fig. 9.2c)
- The elbow crease (Zhouwo) (Fig. 9.3a)
- The Weizhong area on the back of the knee (Fig. 9.3b).

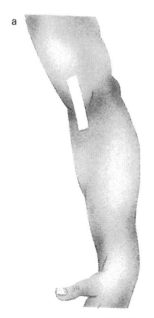
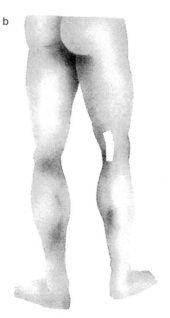

**Fig. 9.3a,b** Friction: locations. **a** Elbow crease **b** Back of the knee.

*Rubbing* (Gua Fa)

Take a small coin or a smooth-edged porcelain soup spoon. Dip them in vegetable oil or water, or coat them with tiger balm.

Rub the area to be treated in one direction only until the skin goes red. Start gently and increase the pressure as you rub. Do not bruise the skin by using too much force.

*Stretching* (Che Sha Fa)

If the objects mentioned above are not available, friction can be performed by stretching. The locations are the same as for rubbing. Hold the edges of the area with your left hand, curl the index and third fingers of your right hand into a hook, dip them in cold water and push down repeatedly, giving the skin a stretch.

The results are the same as for rubbing.

## Indications

- Acute diseases (Shazheng) like cholera, sunstroke:

    Weizhong BL 54, elbow crease, Adam's apple
- Sunstroke (Zhongshu): Taiyang (extra), elbow crease
- Diseases of external origin (Wai Gan): Taiyang (extra), Bladder line on either side of the spine
- Headache: Taiyang (extra)
- Cough and asthma: midline of the thorax; Bladder line
- Sore throat: on both sides of the Adam's apple
- Gastric pain: elbow crease, midline of the thorax
- Abdominal pain: on both sides of the Adam's apple, Weizhong BL 54.

## Precautions

The patient should be comfortable, in a position appropriate to the area being treated.

Start the technique gently and increase the pressure gradually to avoid damaging the skin.

Do not use this technique when there is pain in the spine, or in cases of varicose veins, boil (Chuang), abscess (Ding), or skin infection.

# 10. Qi Gong exercises

Qi Gong, the art of mastering Qi, was originally practised by the Taoists in their search for immortality. It is first mentioned in a Taoist work from the Jin era, the *Catalogue of pure and enlightening beliefs* (265–420 AD).

The medical community first started to show an interest in Qi Gong in 1934, when Tong Hao produced a work entitled *Special treatment for pulmonary tuberculosis: Qi Gong therapy*. After the revolution in 1949, Doctor Liu Gui-zhen founded a sanatorium in Tang Shan where patients were treated with Qi Gong exercise. Since then other sanatoriums of this kind have been built, particularly in Shanghai and Beidahe.

The practice of Qi Gong is based on three principles:

- control of the body,
- regulated breathing,
- mastery of the Shen (spirit).

1. Control of the body is gained through posture: standing, sitting, lying down or walking. Movements can be combined with each of the above. This is expressed in the following axiom:
- stand like a pine tree (Li Ru Song)
- sit like a bell (Zuo Ru Zhong)
- walk like the wind (Xing Ru Feng)
- lie like a bow (Wo Ru Gong).

2. Regulated breathing is achieved either by 'static breathing' i.e. breathing naturally, with calm, slow, gentle and inaudible breaths, or by 'wind breathing', i.e noisy accelerated breathing.

3. Mastery of the spirit is achieved through concentration and meditation exercises.

Different kinds of Qi Gong emerged from the combination of these three areas of training. They vary from the hardest kind, the Qi Gong practised by exponents of the martial arts aiming to develop their physical strength, to the most internal, the Qi Gong of the Taoists seeking a balance between 'non-activity' (Wu Wei) and the 'absence of non-activity' (Bu Wu Wei).

In medicine, the beneficial effects on the metabolism of Qi Gong make it a useful form of therapy for the patient, particularly in chronic disease. It is also beneficial for the practitioner, enhancing his mental and sensory faculties. Qi Gong exercise contributes to the maintenance of good circulation and harmonious balance of Qi and Blood. It regulates the functions of the organs in traditional Chinese medicine from the interior, and is therefore an important element in good health.

The exercises in this chapter come from the kind of Qi Gong known as 'Wind Qi Gong', because the breathing required is noisy. The main aim of these exercises is to develop the practitioner's sensory perception, especially the subtle tactile sensitivity of the fingertips. Qi Gong is therefore recommended as a preliminary to practising needle technique and also benefits the practitioner before a session of acupuncture.

## Practice conditions

Exercise at the same time each day without interruption, preferably on an empty stomach, or a good while after a meal. Practise in the fresh air or in front of an open window in summer, and in a warm but well-ventilated room in winter.

Wear loose and comfortable clothing. To ensure that your feet are flat when exercising, remove shoes with heels and wear slippers. Never exercise barefoot on a cold floor.

For best results keep your mind on the exercise and avoid distraction. Exercise in a quiet place to help your concentration, and try to forget about your worries, thinking only about the movements in the exercise. If performed without concentrating, the exercises will still have a callisthenic effect but the deeper benefits of Qi Gong will be lost.

## Complications

The Qi Gong exercises in this book are not likely to cause complications. The following rules should, however, be followed:

— Practise in a quiet place; stop the session if you are anxious, interrupted, or lose concentration.
— Do not force any of the movements.
— The exercises get progressively harder. Practise each exercise in sequence.

Practising too intensely or in a disorganised way may lead to complications. If respiratory problems develop (sensation of oppression or difficulty in breathing), or if there are abnormal physical sensations or dizziness, stop practising for a while.

## Introductory observations

1. For ease of learning it is better to study the movements of the different phases first. When the sequence of movements flows smoothly the appropriate breathing can be added. For the sake of clarity the exercises have been broken down into phases, but in practice the movements should form an even and harmonious progression, flowing from one phase to the next without interruption until the end of the exercise.
2. Each cycle should be mastered before attempting the next. The practitioner should be able to perform the exercise without running out of breath.
3. Never skip an exercise.
4. If the practice of one cycle proves too difficult, go back a stage, and return to it after a while.
5. Before starting a practice session the practitioner should relax, clear his mind, and put his worries to one side so that he can concentrate on the exercise and reap the maximum benefit from it.

## Cycle I

### Starting position

This position is the same for all the exercises. Stand upright, with your feet parallel, placed as far apart as the width of your shoulders (about 30 cm). You can find this position by standing with your feet together, then moving the heels as far apart as possible with your big toes still touching. Now straighten your feet so they are parallel. Stand with your shoulders lowered, pelvis tilted forwards, legs relaxed, hands on your hips or hanging down.

Clear your mind and try to concentrate on the Dan Tian area (Qihai Ren 6) (Fig. 10.1a).

### Start

Start by emptying your lungs. Bend right over, like a towel on a rope, head hanging down between your arms. Make a loose fist with your hands, thumbs on fingers, wrists relaxed.

The actual exercise starts at this point (Fig. 10.1b).

### Phase 1

Straighten your back, pushing your arms forwards and up until they are vertical. Keep your head between your arms as you come up. They should be stretched but not tense, and the movement should be slow and even.

When the arms are pointing upwards, the head should be straight, eyes looking straight ahead into the distance (Fig. 10.1c).

Move your arms apart, lowering them to your sides in an arc.

When your elbows touch your sides, close your forearms over your chest. Put your fists together on the upper part of the sternum (Fig. 10.1d).

*Breathing.* During phase 1 breathe in once only through the nose from the beginning of the phase to the end, taking a long, even and controlled breath for 20–25 seconds.

Control your breathing by reducing the flow of air in the upper part of the pharynx, so that it makes a noise as it enters the back of the throat. Constrict the passages in the back of your throat to reduce the flow of air and prolong the inhalation. Do not constrict them too much or you will end up snoring.

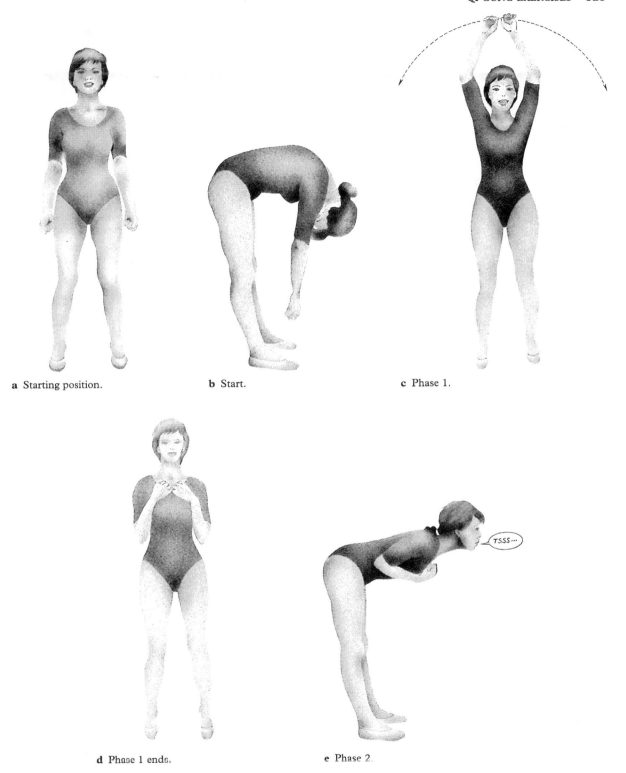

**a** Starting position.          **b** Start.          **c** Phase 1.

**d** Phase 1 ends.          **e** Phase 2.

**Fig. 10.1a–e**   Qi Gong Cycle I.

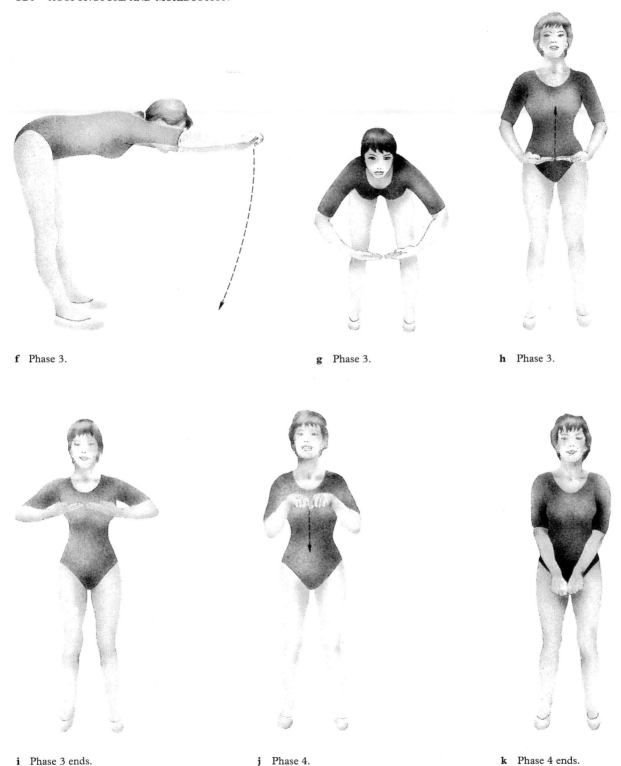

f   Phase 3.

g   Phase 3.

h   Phase 3.

i   Phase 3 ends.

j   Phase 4.

k   Phase 4 ends.

**Fig. 10.1f–k**   Qi Gong Cycle I.

Practical advice: if you are unable to prolong the inhalation for the duration of the phase, hold your breath until the movement is completed. Practise matching your breath to the length of the movement so that you can master it as quickly as possible.

### Phase 2

Keep your arms in the same position.

Bend down at the waist quite briskly so that your torso is parallel to the floor. Keep looking straight ahead, pushing your chin out to free the trachea (Fig. 10.1e).

*Breathing.* Breathe out through the mouth. Bring your teeth together and put your tongue behind them. Push your breath out forcefully, making a 'Tsss' hissing sound like a rattlesnake.

The air is compressed throughout the exhalation by the position of the tongue against the teeth. Half open the mouth to finish, expelling the remaining air abruptly with a '. . .Sss'.

### Phase 3

Open your hands, stretching your fingers outwards, and extend your arms forwards parallel to the ground as if you were about to dive. Bring them out to the sides then lower them, rounding them as if encircling a huge imaginary ball resting on the ground (Fig. 10.1f).

Bring your hands together on the ground, palms open and facing up with the tips of your third fingers touching. Keep your torso parallel to the ground, arms curved in a big circle (Fig. 10.1g).

Straighten your back to the vertical whilst lifting the imaginary ball of air along your legs. Your hands do not move independently; they come up as you straighten your back. The ball of air should stay the same size. Keep your palms flat; do not curve them like serving spoons (Fig. 10.1h).

When your torso is back in the upright position, start to move your hands further up, gradually crushing the ball of air. Stop your hands, which should still be flat and open, level with your breast, ulnar border towards the nipples. Hold your shoulders down, elbows free and in the lateral plane, and look straight ahead (Fig. 10.1i).

*Breathing.* Breathe in through the nose. Breathing should be slow and controlled (in the same way as

phase 1), and last for the entire length of the movement.

### Phase 4

Close your fists and turn them over so that the palms are underneath, thumbs touching, as if holding the brush of an upside-down broomstick (Fig. 10.1j).

Keeping your posture straight, push your fists abruptly down, as if forcing the brush down the broomstick. This should cause a shock which travels along the arm, up the back of the neck to the head, which remains straight (Fig. 10.1k).

*Breathing.* Breathe out rapidly through the nose. The air should be expelled from the nose with the same speed, sound and compression as if you were blowing it. As you cannot hold your nose, the action of the fingers is replaced by contraction of the nostrils and lateral muscles of the nose (myrtiform muscles). Some mucus may be discharged as you breathe out.

Exercise ends.

Repeat the whole exercise exactly 6 times in a row. This sequence of 6 exercises constitutes Cycle I.

If possible, practise Cycle I once in the morning and once in the evening. Continue for a month before moving on to Cycle II.

### Observations

1. During initial training, you may experience some visual disturbances, feel dizzy, or even faint. If these problems are severe, start off doing the exercises sitting down. Sit on the edge of a chair with your feet parallel and positioned as far apart as the width of your shoulders.

2. If you feel out of breath at the end of the exercise, repeat phases 3 and 4 two or three times in a row.

## Cycle II

### Phase 1

Go back to the starting position: bent right over, with your head hanging down between your arms. Keep your hands in a loose fist, thumbs on fingers, wrists relaxed (Fig. 10.2a).

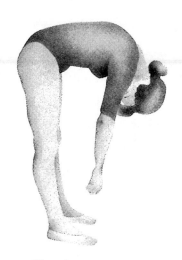

**a**  Phase 1.

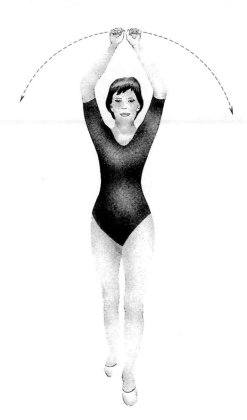

**b**  Phase 1.

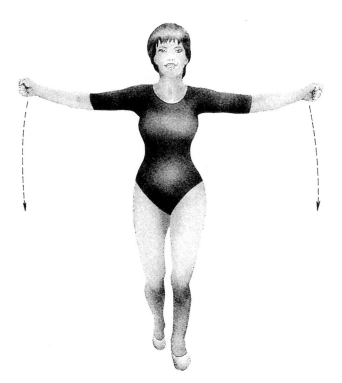

**c**  Phase 1.

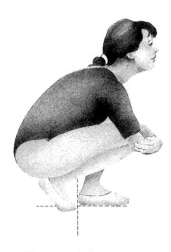

**d**  Phase 1 and Phase 2 end.

**Fig. 10.2a–d**  Qi Gong Cycle II.

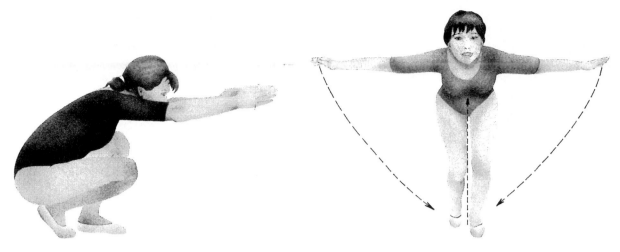

e Phase 3.

f Phase 3.

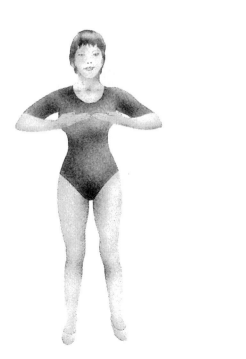

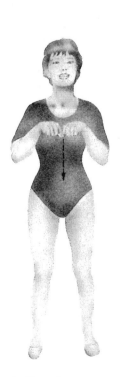

g Phase 3 ends.

h Phase 4.

**Fig. 10.2e–h** Qi Gong Cycle II.

In the same way as in the first exercise, straighten your back, pushing your arms forwards and up until they are vertical. Keep your head between your arms as you come up. Arms should be stretched but not tense, and the movement should be slow and even. When your arms are pointing upwards, your head should be straight, eyes looking straight ahead into the distance.

As you move your arms apart and lower them in an arc, raise your left foot and bring it forwards, putting it down with the heel level with the tip of your right foot. Keep both feet straight, resting on either side of an imaginary line running along the medial edge of each foot (Fig. 10.2b, c).

At the same time crouch down, keeping your left foot flat and raising the heel of your right foot. As you crouch down, sit on the heel of your right foot and put your arms around your knees.

When you have put your arms around your knees, your left knee should fit into the crook of your left elbow, and your right knee into the crook of your right elbow. If possible, your elbows should be cupped in your hands (Fig. 10.2d).

Keep your head straight when you are crouching down, chin extended to free the trachea, eyes looking straight ahead into the distance.

*Breathing.* Breathe in. Inhale in exactly the same way as in Cycle I, Phase 1: Breathe in once through the nose in a long, even and controlled breath for 20–25 seconds.

### Phase 2

Remain in the crouching position.

*Breathing.* Breathe out through the mouth. Push the air out in the same way as in Cycle I, Phase 2: bring your teeth together and put your tongue behind them. Push your breath out forcefully, making a hissing sound like a rattlesnake. Half open the mouth to finish, expelling the remaining air abruptly.

If the exhalation is performed properly, you should be able to feel a contraction in the lumbar area as the remaining air is expelled.

### Phase 3

As you begin to stand up, raise your hips and take

hold of the imaginary ball of air in the same way as in Cycle I, Phase 3 (Fig. 10.2e, f).

Slowly straighten up whilst putting your left foot back in place parallel to your right foot. Continue raising the ball with your arms as far as your nipples, in the same way as in Cycle I (Fig. 10.2g).

*Breathing.* Controlled inhalation through the nose, as in Cycle I, Phase 1.

### Phase 4

The movement is the same as Cycle I, Phase 4: close your fists and turn them over so that the palms are underneath, thumbs touching (Fig. 10.2h). Keeping your posture straight, push your fists down abruptly.

*Breathing.* The same as in Cycle I, Phase 4: breathe out rapidly through the nose, as if blowing it.

Exercise ends.

Cycle II consists of repeating the exercise 6 times.

If possible, practise Cycle I followed by Cycle II once in the morning and once in the evening. Continue for a month before moving on to Cycle III.

## Cycle III

### Starting position

Stand in the initial starting position: feet parallel, spaced as far apart as the width of your shoulders, pelvis tilted forwards. Keep your centre of gravity low, with your weight distributed evenly between both feet.

### Start

Relax your shoulders, and make a tight fist with each hand, thumbs on fingers, and rest them on your hips. Move your fists backwards until the knuckle of the index finger is pressing into the hollow of the kidneys, in the angle formed between the iliac crests and the spinal muscles.

The exercise starts when the fists are in place (Fig. 10.3a, posterior view, 10.3b, anterior view).

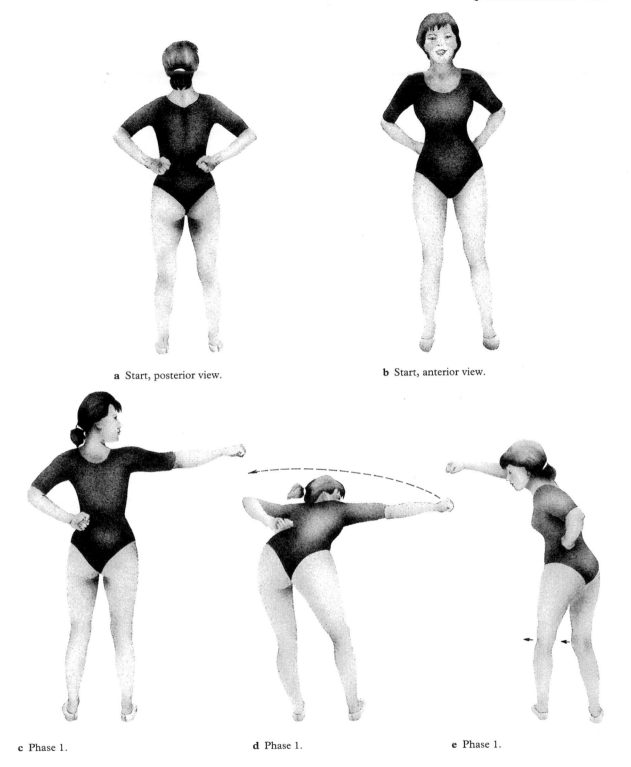

**a** Start, posterior view.

**b** Start, anterior view.

**c** Phase 1.

**d** Phase 1.

**e** Phase 1.

**Fig. 10.3a–e** Qi Gong Cycle III.

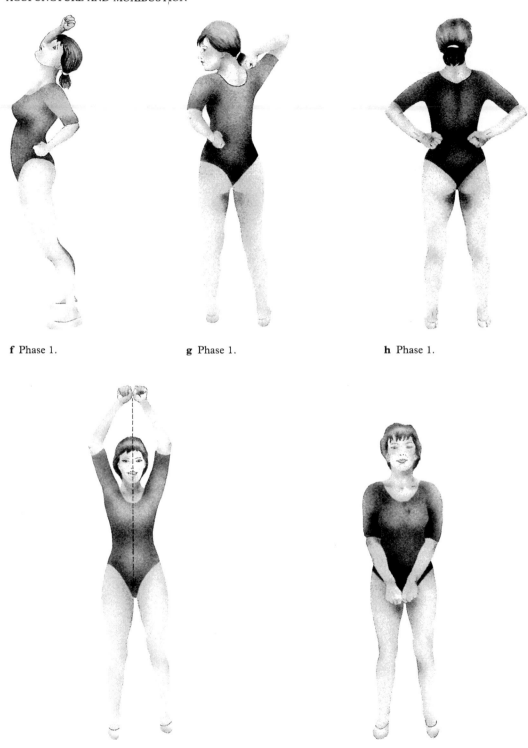

f Phase 1.                g Phase 1.                h Phase 1.

i Phase 2.                          j Phase 2 ends.

**Fig. 10.3f–j**   Qi Gong Cycle III.

*Phase 1*

Leave your left fist in position. Keeping your right fist closed, extend your right arm to the side, turning your head to the right and fixing your gaze on the right fist (Fig. 10.3c).

In one movement bend your right knee and tilt your torso about 45° to the right. Lower your head slightly so that your arm is at the same height as your ear. Keep looking at the right fist. Your left leg should remain extended, and both feet should be flat on the ground (Fig. 10.3d).

From this position flex your right knee and torso as far as possible and start a circular movement to the left. As you rotate, your weight should move gradually from one leg to the other. At the end of the movement the body should be flexed 45° to the left, your left leg flexed and right leg extended. Your right arm remains extended level with the ear and follows the movement. Keep looking at the right fist all the time (Fig. 10.3e).

Continue rotating your torso, leaning as far back as possible, extending the neck backwards. At the same time bend your arm back to bring your forearm behind the back of your neck (Fig. 10.3f).

When your torso is back in the sagittal plane straighten up and put your legs back in the starting position. Slide your right fist forwards along your neck and down the side of your torso (Fig. 10.3g), then put it back on your hip in the starting position (Fig. 10.3h).

Starting from the left, perform the opposite movement.

The two movements together constitute one sequence, which is performed three times.

*Breathing.* Breathe in through the nose. Breathe in once only, with one even and controlled breath in the course of the entire phase.

*Phase 2*

Move your fists away from your hips and lift them up laterally in an arc. Join them over your head, thumbs touching (Fig. 10.3i), then push them down quickly and forcefully in a pumping movement as in Cycle II, Phase 4 (Fig. 10.3j).

*Breathing.* Breathe out through the nose. Start to breathe out when your fists have met about your head and are starting to come down. Expel the air noisily, rapidly and forcefully, as if blowing your nose (see above, Cycle I, Phase 4).

Exercise ends.

Cycle III consists of repeating the exercise 6 times in a row.

If possible, practise Cycles I, II, and III once in the morning and once in the evening. Continue for a month before moving on to Cycle IV.

### Observations

1. At the end of the cycle the movement should have been performed 18 times from the right and 18 times from the left.
2. Beginners often experience difficulties making the inhalation last up to the end of Phase 1. If this is the case, when your lungs are full hold your breath till the end of the phase and breathe out once you have completed the 6 movements. With training your breathing will improve and you will be able to extend the inhalation until you have finished the movements.
3. Between each exercise get your breath back by performing Phases 3 and 4 of Cycle I, 2 or 3 times in a row.
4. If holding your breath with your lungs full proves to be too painful go back to practising Cycle II, and do not attempt Cycle III until you have enough breath.

### Cycle IV

From Cycle IV onwards the focus on the Qihai Ren 6 area becomes more intense, and a Qi Gong belt should be worn to support the Dan Tian area and keep it warm.

### Making the belt

The belt is made of a strip of strong cotton, folded over to make it double thickness. For women it should be 7 cm wide, and for men between 8 and 9 cm. It should be 90–150 cm in length, depending on the size of the waist. The total length should be equal to approximately one and a half times the size of the waist. Attach two or three braided cords to each end so that the belt can be fastened at the front. Reinforce the middle 20 cm or thereabouts with a few rows of stitching.

## Wearing the belt

The middle of the reinforced part goes just below the navel, on the upper part of the lower abdomen. The centre of the belt covers the Qihai Ren 6 point, or the lower Dan Tian.

Cross the cords over behind your back, bring them round to the front, and tie them together directly over the Qihai point. If the knot is placed inaccurately the organs may be damaged in the long term.

## Starting position

Put on the belt, then go into the standing position, feet parallel, pelvis tilted forwards, with your weight distributed evenly between the feet.

## Start

Relax your shoulders, make a tight fist with each hand, thumbs on fingers. Put your fists on your hips, then move them backwards into the hollow of your kidneys, as in Cycle III. The exercise starts when your fists are in place (Fig. 10.4a).

## Phase 1

Leave your left fist in position. Keeping your right fist closed, extend your right arm to the side, turning your head to the right and fixing your gaze on the right fist (Fig. 10.4b).

Bend your arm and bring your fist in front of your face, following it with your eyes. Continue the movement, bringing your fist round as far as possible to above your left shoulder (Fig. 10.4c), then move it back in front of you, following it with your eyes all the time (Fig. 10.4d).

The hips should not move at all during the movement. As your fist passes your face, only the torso pivots to the left, returning to face the front at the same time as your fist.

Phase 1 ends.

*Breathing.* Breathe in once only, with one slow, even and controlled breath in the course of the entire phase. When you finish breathing in, swallow some saliva whilst pushing your hips forwards and pushing the air against the knot of the belt. Now let out a tiny breath of air from the mouth, as if spitting out a fragment of food stuck on the tip of your tongue.

## Phase 2

Move your right arm in a huge arc (Fig. 10.4e) and touch the tip of the lateral malleolus with the back of the fist (the knuckle of your third finger) (Fig. 10.4f).

Lift your arm high above your head for this movement and flex your torso *laterally*. Keep your right leg extended and bend your left knee.

Without pausing, open your hand and bring it into pronation. Straighten up till your torso is vertical and at the same time move your elbow backwards so that the open hand is level with the hips. Keep your hand open, fingers together, hand extended as far as possible so it is at right angles to the plane of the forearm (Fig. 10.4g).

Phase 2 ends.

*Breathing.* Hold your breath throughout the movement.

## Phase 3

Move your head 45° to the right. Without changing the position of your hand, extend your arm forwards slowly in the direction of your gaze, moving it with little jerks as if pushing something very heavy (Fig. 10.4h).

Movement ends.

*Breathing.* Contract your nostrils and breathe out slowly and forcefully through the nose, prolonging the exhalation until your arm is fully extended. This is the same kind of exhalation practised in Cycle I, Phase 4, but performed slowly.

Bring your right fist back to the hollow of your kidney, then do the inverse exercise with the left arm.

Extend both arms, lean forwards and finish the cycle with Phases 3 and 4 of Cycle I (Fig. 10.1 f–k).

Cycle IV consists of repeating the exercise 6 times from the right and 6 times from the left.

If possible, practise Cycles I, II, III and IV once in the morning and once in the evening. Continue for a month before moving on to Cycle V.

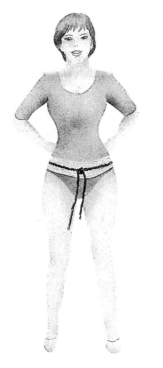

**a** Starting position.

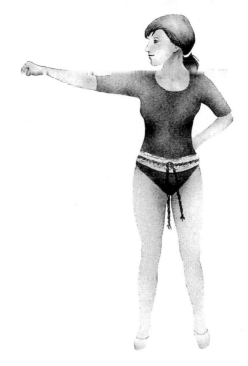

**b** Phase 1.

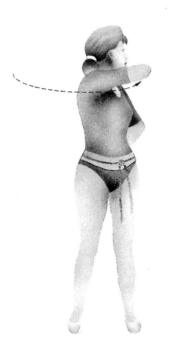

**c** Phase 1.

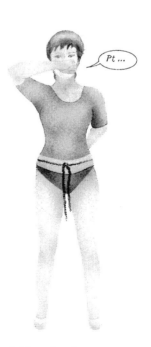

**d** Phase 1 ends.

**Fig. 10.4a–d** Qi Gong Cycle IV.

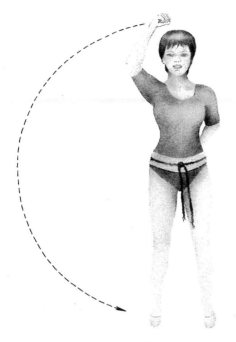

**e** Phase 2.

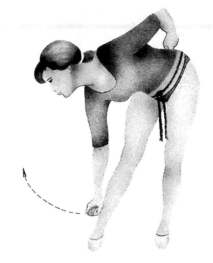

**f** Phase 2.

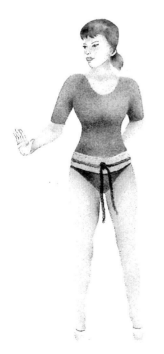

**g** Phase 2.

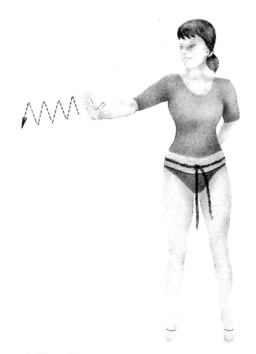

**h** Phase 3.

**Fig. 10.4e–h** Qi Gong Cycle IV.

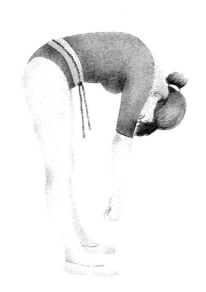

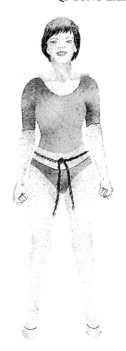

**a** Start.

**b** Phase 1.

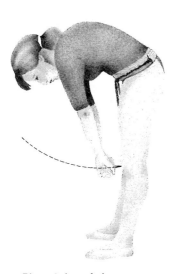

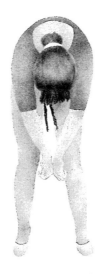

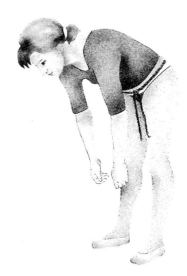

**c** Phase 2, lateral view.

**d** Phase 2, anterior view.

**e** Phase 4.

**Fig. 10.5a–e** Qi Gong Cycle V.

## Cycle V

Put on the Qi Gong belt.

### *Starting position*

Stand straight with your feet parallel, hips tilted forwards, concentrating on the Dan Tian.

### *Start*

Bend over as in Cycle I, head hanging down between your arms. Make a loose fist with your hands, wrists relaxed (Fig. 10.5a).

### *Phase 1*

As in Cycle I, straighten up slowly, pushing your arms as far forwards as possible. Join your fists together to make a circle above your head, then let your arms hang down by your sides, with your hands still gently clenched (Fig. 10.5b).

Phase 1 ends.

*Breathing.* As in Cycle IV. Take a slow, even and controlled breath, tilting your hips forwards and pushing the air against the knot of the belt. Finish by expelling a tiny breath of air from the mouth.

### *Phase 2*

Lean forwards and put your fists back to back. Place them on your knees over the patellae. Round your back and bring your shoulders forwards and inwards (Fig. 10.5c, lateral view, Fig. 10.5d, anterior view).

*Breathing.* Hold your breath.

### *Phase 3*

Contract your anus and try to keep it raised.

At the same time make your head tremble imperceptibly from right to left, with powerful progressive and rhythmic contractions of the two sternocleidomastoid muscles. Continue these contractions for 10 seconds.

*Breathing.* As you are already holding your breath you will only be able to take in a little more air, but try to inhale some more (slow and controlled breathing), persevering for the 10 seconds of the phase.

### *Phase 4*

Completely relax and let your arms drop (Fig. 10.5e).

*Breathing.* Breathe out forcefully through the mouth.

Continue with Phases 3 and 4 of Cycle I.

Exercise ends.

Repeat this exercise 6 times.

When you have completed Cycle V, continue practising the entire series of cycles regularly, preferably twice a day.

### *Observations*

1. Do not be in a hurry to move on from one cycle to the next. It is important to master the movements and breathing patterns of each one.

2. Exercise calmly and slowly. All 5 cycles together should take between 20 and 30 minutes.

3. If you are interrupted during exercise and are unable to regain your tranquillity and concentration, it is better to stop.

### *Effectiveness*

Practised regularly these exercises will sharpen your tactile sensitivity, and refine the subtlety of your touch. They will also increase the power of your concentration and clear your mind.

Your commitment will be richly rewarded.

# Appendix I. Training programme

This book offers numerous descriptions of different techniques of training. Some of these are designed to increase manual dexterity or enhance the sensitivity of the fingers. Others are designed for therapeutic purposes, but must be regularly practised before they can be mastered and used.

Learning all these techniques requires a logical sequence of study. Below is a training programme, which has been conceived to run over a period of 10 months, corresponding roughly to the academic year. The programme is broken up into five blocks of two months, in the course of which every exercise and technique is covered in succession.

Each block has been carefully designed so that the whole programme provides a sound training for the average person. The individual student can use it as a blueprint, moving forward at his own pace, but two principles should be borne in mind:

1. Master each exercise completely before moving on to the next one.

2. Practise regularly and constantly. Any lapse in practice will set you back.

The student should have no illusions about learning proper needle technique; it cannot be done quickly, or without a lot of effort. One thing is beyond doubt: the prize for perseverance is that every step towards mastering needle insertion and manipulation will immediately manifest itself in better therapeutic results.

## Frequency and duration of practice

For best results the student should practise morning and evening. To start with the various exercises will take between 10 and 15 minutes. Later on they will take considerably longer, as new exercises are added.

## BLOCK I — Months 1 and 2

Each session consists of:

- Qi Gong
- ball exercises
- polishing the needle
- practising on the cushion.

### Qi gong

Practise Cycle I each session.

### Ball exercises

Practise with the golf balls: 1 minute per hand in month 1, then 2 minutes per hand in month 2.

### Polishing the needle

Practise polishing the needle for 2 minutes per session. Pull your thumb towards you as you move the needle down, rotating it anti-clockwise.

### Practising on the cushion

During each session:

a. Practise inserting the needle for 2 minutes.
b. Spend 5 minutes practising the first two techniques:
1. reinforcing by lifting and thrusting (Ti Cha)
2. reducing by lifting and thrusting (Ti Cha).

## BLOCK II — Months 3 and 4

Each session consists of:

- Qi Gong
- ball exercises
- polishing the needle
- practising on the cushion.

### Qi Gong

Practise Cycle I followed by Cycle II each session. Always practise the cycles in the correct order.

### Ball exercises

Practise with the golf balls: 5 minutes per hand, or 5 series of 100 uninterrupted revolutions.

### Polishing the needle

Practise for 3 minutes altogether.

For the first 2 minutes practise pulling your thumb towards you while thrusting the needle in, rotating it anti-clockwise.

Reverse the movement for the third minute. Extend your thumb whilst thrusting the needle in, rotating it clockwise.

### Practising on the cushion

During each session:

a. Practise inserting the needle for 2 minutes.
b. Spend 5 minutes revising the first two techniques and learn the following:
3. reinforcing by rotation (Nian Zhuan)
4. reducing by rotation (Nian Zhuan)
5. balancing (Ping Bu Ping Xie).

## BLOCK III — Months 5 and 6

Each session consists of:

- Qi Gong
- ball exercises
- stick exercises
- polishing the needle
- practising on the cushion.

### Qi Gong

Practise Cycles I, II and III in sequence.

If holding your breath is too difficult when you first start Cycle III, leave it for a while and come back to it only when your breathing is strong enough.

### Ball exercises

Replace the golf balls with the round stones. These balls are heavier than golf balls. Exercise for 2 minutes per hand in month 5. Increase gradually to 5 minutes or 5 series of 100 revolutions in month 6.

### Stick exercises

Practise with one hand at a time, starting with your right hand.

Start with 1 minute per hand in month 5, progressing to 2 minutes per hand in month 6.

This exercise puts a lot of strain on the elbow. If you begin to get cramps stop practising for a while, then gradually start again.

### Polishing the needle

Practise for 4 minutes. For the first 2 minutes rotate the needle anti-clockwise and for the last 2 minutes rotate it clockwise.

### Practising on the cushion

a. Spend 2 minutes practising oblique and horizontal needle insertion.
b. Spend 5 minutes revising the techniques already learned and add the following complex manipulations:
6. lighting the fire on the mountain (Shao Shan Huo)
7. coolness from heaven (Tou Tian Liang)
8. reinforcing by obtaining sensations of heat
9. reducing by obtaining sensations of cold.

These manipulations use basic movements already studied in the simple techniques, so they should be easy to master. However, to carry out the complex techniques properly, the student must be able to perform the simple ones with ease.

## BLOCK IV — Months 7 and 8

Each session consists of:

- Qi Gong
- ball exercises
- stick exercises
- polishing the needle
- practising on the cushion.

### Qi Gong

Practise Cycles I, II, III and IV in sequence.

### Ball exercises

Replace the rounded stones with the steel balls, which are heavier still.

Practise for 2 minutes per hand in month 7, progressing to 5 minutes or 5 series of 100 revolutions per hand in month 8.

### Stick exercises

Start with 3 minutes per hand in month 7, then 4 minutes per hand in month 8.

### Polishing the needle

Practise for 4 minutes, alternating the direction of rotation and counting the number of times you thrust the needle in. Thrust the needle in 9 times or a multiple of 9 times, extending your thumb as the needle goes in, then thrust the needle in 6 times or a multiple of 6 times, pulling your thumb towards you as the needle goes in.

### Practising on the cushion

a. Spend 2 minutes inserting the needle (perpendicular, oblique and horizontal insertion). Do not confine yourself to the top of the cushion: try needling the front and the back as well.

b. Spend 5 minutes revising the techniques already learned (1–9), and add the following:
10. green tortoise seeks the point (Cang Gui Tan Xue)
11. flying away (Fei)
12. green dragon swings his tail (Cang Long Yao Wei).

### BLOCK V — Months 9 and 10

Each session consists of:

- Qi Gong
- ball exercises
- stick exercises
- bottle exercises
- polishing the needle
- practising on the cushion.

### Qi Gong

Add Cycle V and practise the entire series regularly each session.

### Ball exercises

Continue practising with the steel balls for 5 minutes per hand, or start to use musical balls (Chinese exercise balls).

### Stick exercises

Increase your practice time to 5 minutes per hand.

### Bottle exercises

Practise for 1 minute to start with, increasing to a maximum of 5 minutes.

### Polishing the needle

Practise polishing the needle for 5 minutes, alternating the direction of rotation and counting the number of times you thrust the needle in: thrust 9 times or a multiple of 9 times, or 6 times or a multiple of 6 times.

### Practising on the cushion

a. Practise insertion for 2 minutes. Learn 'insertion into tough skin' and 'one-handed insertion'.

b. Revise the techniques already covered (1–12), and learn the remainder:
13. white tiger shakes his head (Bai Hu Yao Tou)
14. Yin hidden in Yang (Yang Zhong Yin Yin Fa)
15. Yang hidden in Yin (Yin Zhong Yin Yang Fa)
16. dragon and tiger come to blows (Long Hu Jiao Zhan).

## OVERVIEW OF TRAINING PROGRAMME

| Block | Qi Gong | Balls | Stick | Bottle | Polishing the needle | Needle techniques |
|---|---|---|---|---|---|---|
| I | Cycle I | Golf 1–2 minutes per hand | — | — | 2 minutes | Insertion 2 minutes. Techniques 1 and 2 |
| II | Cycle I, II | Golf 5 minutes per hand | — | — | 3 minutes | Insertion 2 minutes. Techniques 1–5 |
| III | Cycle I, II, III | Stone 2–5 minutes per hand | 1–2 minutes per hand | — | 4 minutes | Insertion 2 minutes. Techniques 1–9 |
| IV | Cycle I, II, III, IV | Steel 2–5 minutes per hand | 3–4 minutes per hand | — | 4 minutes | Insertion 2 minutes. Techniques 1–12 |
| V | Cycle I, II, III, IV, V | Steel or musical 5 minutes per hand | 5 minutes per hand | 1–5 minutes maximum | 5 minutes | Insertion 2 minutes. All techniques. |

# Appendix II. Needle techniques: revision table

| Name | Aim | Method |
|------|-----|--------|
| 1. Reinforcing by lifting and thrusting<br>Ti Cha | Reinforcing | Thrust forcefully, withdraw gently. |
| 2. Reducing by lifting and thrusting<br>Ti Cha | Reducing | Withdraw forcefully, thrust gently. |
| 3. Reinforcing by rotation<br>Nian Zhuan | Reinforcing | Rotation through a small angle, pulling your thumb towards you 9 times or a multiple of 9 times. |
| 4. Reducing by rotation<br>Nian Zhuan | Reducing | Rotation through 180° to 360°, extending your thumb 6 times or a multiple of 6 times. |
| 5. Balancing<br>Ping Bu Ping Xie | Equal Reinforcing and Reducing<br>Obtaining Qi | Push in whilst rotating, pulling your thumb towards you. Withdraw whilst rotating in the opposite direction. |
| 6. Lighting the fire on the mountain<br>Shao Shan Huo | Reinforcing<br>Obtaining Qi<br>Sensations of heat | Reinforcing rotation on 3 levels, 9 times on each level. |
| 7. Coolness from heaven<br>Tou Tian Liang | Reducing<br>Sensations of cold | Reducing rotation on 3 levels, 6 times on each level. |
| 8. Reinforcing by obtaining sensations of heat | Reinforcing<br>Obtaining sensations of heat | Reinforcing rotation on 3 levels. Entwine fibres around needle, scratch, unwind and remove. |
| 9. Reducing by obtaining sensations of cold | Reducing<br>Obtaining sensations of cold | Reducing rotation on 3 levels. Entwine fibres around needle, scratch, unwind and remove. |
| 10. Green tortoise seeks the point<br>Cang Gui Tan Xue | Reinforcing<br>Searching for and obtaining Qi | Thrust then lift needle whilst moving it in a circle in the vertical plane. |
| 11. Flying away<br>Fei | Reinforcing or Reducing | Pinch needle between thumb and index finger. Flick away either thumb or index finger, whilst opening hand. |
| 12. Green dragon swings his tail<br>Cang Long Yao Wei | Moving Qi<br>Reinforcing | Curve handle over left index finger and shake as if plying a scull. |
| 13. White tiger shakes his head<br>Bai Hu Yao Tou | Moving Qi<br>Reducing | Swing needle gently over index finger then in other direction. |

| Name | Aim | Method |
|------|-----|--------|
| 14. Yin hidden in Yang<br>Yang Zhong Yin Yin Fa | Reinforcing with element of Reducing | Thrust forcefully to half depth of point, then reinforce with Ti Cha (9 times). Thrust gently to full depth and reduce with Ti Cha (6 times). |
| 15. Yang hidden in Yin<br>Yin Zhong Yin Yang Fa | Reducing with element of Reinforcing | Thrust gently to full depth of point, then reduce with Ti Cha (6 times). Withdraw to half depth and reinforce with Ti Cha (9 times). |
| 16. Dragon and tiger come to blows<br>Long Hu Jiao Zhan | Reinforcing and Reducing Treats Cold and Heat, balances Yin and Yang | On 3 arm Yang, 3 leg Yin and Ren Mai, rotate 9 times to reinforce, then 6 times to reduce. On 3 arm Yin, 3 leg Yang and Du Mai, rotate 6 times to reduce, then 9 times to reinforce. |

# Bibliography

Li Tianyuan: Personal correspondence.

Li Wenhui, He Baoyi: *Shiyong Zhenjiu Xue*. Renmin Weisheng Chubanshe, Beijing, 1981.

*Ling Shu Jing: Ma Huantai* edition, 1806.

*Ling Shu Jing Jiaoshi*: 2 volumes, annotated by He Bei Xue Yuan. Renmin Weisheng Chubanshe, Beijing, 1982.

Lu Shouyan and Zhu Rugong: *Zhenjiu Xue Xicong*. Shanghai Kexue Jishu Chubanshe, Shanghai, 1959.

*Mei Hua Zhen Liao Fa*: Zhongyi Yanjiu Guang An Men Yiyuan. Renmin Weisheng Chubanshe, Beijing, 1973.

*Nan Jing Yishi*: Nanjing Zhongyi Xueyuan. Shanghai Kexue Jishu Chubanshe, Shanghai , 1961.

*The Second national symposium on acupuncture and moxibustion and acupuncture anesthesia. Abstracts*. Beijing China, 1984: No. 108 p. 105, No. 109 p. 105, 106, No. 110 p. 106–108, No. 111 p. 108, No. 112 p. 109, 110, No. 113 p. 110, 111, No. 114 p. 111, No. 115 p. 112, No. 116 p. 112, 113, No. 119 p. 114, 115, No. 120 p. 115, 116, No. 121 p. 116, 117.

Xi Yongjiang: *Zhen Fa Jiu Fa Xue*. Shanghai Kexue Jishu Chubanshe, Shanghai, 1983.

Yang Jizhou: *Zhen Jiu Da Cheng*, 1601. Renmin Weisheng Chubanshe edition, Beijing, 1973.

Yang Jizhou: *Zhen Jiu Da Cheng*, 1601. Fonds Soubeiran, 1843 edition.

Yang Mingyuan: *Jianming Zhenjiu Xue*. Heilongjiang Renmin Chubanshe, Harbin, 1981.

Zheng Kuishan: *Zhen Jiu Ji Jin*. Gansu Renmin Chubanshe, Lanzhou, 1978.

*Zhenjiu Xue*: Chengdu Zhongyi Xueyuan. Sichuan Renmin Chubanshe, Chengdu, 1981.

*Zhenjiu Xue*: Nanjing Zhongyi Xueyuan. Jiangsu Renmin Chubanshe, Nanjing, 1957.

*Zhenjiu Xue*: Nanjing Zhongyi Xueyuan. Shanghai Kexue Jishu Chubanshe, Shanghai, 1978.

*Zhenjiu Xue*: Shanghai Zhongyi Xueyuan. Renmin Weisheng Chubanshe, Shanghai, 1974.

*Zhenjiu Xue Jianbian*: Zhongyi Yanjiu Yuan. Renmin Weisheng Chubanshe, Beijing, 1957.

Zhong Meiquan: *Zhongguo Meihua Zhen*. Renmin Weisheng Chubanshe, Beijing, 1982.

# Index

Edwards Brothers Inc.
Ann Arbor MI. USA
August 17, 2011